I AIN'T DONE
LIVING
YET

I AIN'T DONE LIVING YET

A CORONAVIRUS SURVIVOR MEMOIR

MARQUES A. EASON, ESQ.

I AIN'T DONE LIVING YET

A Coronavirus Survivor Memoir

November Media Publishing

Copyright © 2021 Marques A. Eason, Esq.

For permission requests, write to the author, addressed "attention: Marques A. Eason, Esq." at the email address below.

meason@marqueseasonlaw.com

Ordering information: special discounts are available on quantity purchases by corporations, associations, and others. For details, contact the author at the email address above.

Printed in the United States of America
Published & Produced by November Media Publishing

All Scriptures quotations, unless otherwise indicated, are taken from the New American Standard Bible (NASB), King James Version, CJB, Voice, RSV, EXB.

ISBN-13: 978-1-7354542-8-3

TABLE OF CONTENTS

PAST

PRESENT

FUTURE

DEDICATION

First and foremost, I give honor to almighty GOD. I battled a beast, and GOD guided me to the other side with nothing more than a battle scar. GOD's mercy and grace is the reason I am still alive today. GOD is the reason why I survived the coronavirus ("COVID-19"). GOD is the reason why I came home, and He is the reason I have the courage and the motivation to tell my COVID-19 story. GOD spared my life so that I could fulfill the purpose He has in mind for me. I am both a living witness and one of God's miracles, and for that I am forever grateful.

Second, I dedicate this book to my mother, Barbara Eason-Watkins. GOD could not have blessed me with a better mother. My mother has been my pillar of strength throughout this whole ordeal. Despite what she was going through internally, she had the strength to speak to the doctors daily, send regular reports to those closest to me, while still being responsible for running a school district in Indiana. As strong as my mother was during this period of uncertainty, Tiffany's uplifting spirit and presence, made an otherwise challenging time less difficult. My mother galvanized a network of prayer warriors, consisting of friends, family, and people that I did not even know, who spent countless hours while I was sedated, praying for my recovery. I would be remised if I did not thank Dr. Irvin B. Watkins ("Irv"), my stepfather, for also taking care of my mother, as he always does, but even more so during an uncertain time where it was unclear whether I would survive my ordeal with COVID-19.

Third, I dedicate this book to my daughter, Amber Eldridge. Like my mother, Amber was a trooper in her own right. I have two daughters, Amber, and Vivian. Vivian and I have a challenging and troubled relationship. I had not seen her, or my grandbaby, Blake, in the three years prior to my COVID-19 experience, and I have not heard from her since. However, Amber, along with her mother, Karen, called the hospital while I was intubated and received daily updates from the nurses. Amber sent daily gut-wrenching text messages to me that literally broke my heart and hers was the first voice that I heard when I woke up from being sedated. As did my mother, both Amber and Karen also informed me of what I had gone through each day prior to waking up from sedation—things I never knew before my mother shared her daily text messages from her prayer network.

Fourth, I want to thank the doctors and nurses, and all the medical and professional staff at the University of Chicago main campus hospital for their skilled expertise and hard work in helping me defeat the coronavirus, in particular Dr. Daniel Ash, Dr. Jennifer Wolf (my orthopedic hand surgeon), Russell and Barbara (my occupational therapists), and the Ingalls Memorial Rehabilitation staff, especially Kevin

Vicari (my physical therapist while in rehab). GOD certainly blessed me with the best to make sure that I came out of this alive. I have been meaning to reach out to each of them individually to thank them. I still plan to do so, but would like to acknowledge them, in case they may be reading this, and let them know that without them, I have no survival story to tell.

Fifth, this book is dedicated to my brother and best friend—the late, great, Otha Smith Jr (1974-2018), and my sister, Nicole Marie Lazarus (1978-2002). Otha died suddenly in his sleep on September 8th, 2018. I call him the "Big O in the Sky". O left us way too soon. He was always a friend and brother to Kris and me, as well to the group of friends that to this day we affectionately call "CREW". As scary and uncertain as my ordeal was, I had no doubt that GOD sent O as an angel to watch over me and make sure that I survived and lived to share this testimony.

Nicole was killed in a road rage incident in June 2002. Her killer, Latashia Porter, was convicted of first-degree murder, after a judge in a bench trial, found that Porter intentionally hit the van being driven by her boyfriend, who apparently had two other women in the vehicle with him. The boyfriend's van spun out of control into a head on collision with Nicole's vehicle, killing her instantly. Porter was sentenced to 35 years in prison and is currently an inmate at Logan Correctional Center in Lincoln, Illinois. **#UnnecessaryCollateralDamage**

Sixth, this book is dedicated to Laurentia Brooks, my beautiful friend and ("birthday twin"), with whom I am honored to share the same birthdate of March 10th with each year. During our conversation, while I was in rehab, she told me to *"Get totally well sir! We Ain't Done Living Yet!"* Little did she know at the time that her words inspired the title of this book, ***"I Ain't Done Living Yet!"***

Finally, Gregg Garfield, 54, a native of Southern California, and otherwise known as "Patient Zero". He was the first known U.S. Coronavirus patient who spent 64 days total in the ICU, and 41 days total sedated on a ventilator. Gregg had a 1% chance of survival but pulled through. Gregg and 12 others went on a ski trip to Italy, just as the virus was making its initial wave through Northern Italy. All 13 people in his group caught the virus, but Gregg's health worsened over time. Like me, Gregg survived and has plans to hit the ski slopes once again. I first read his story on People's Magazine website, after my mother brought it to my attention. He was gracious enough to speak with me on Facebook. We shared stories, including the hallucinations, and otherwise, weird dreams that we both had while under sedation, as well as other similar health challenges and experiences. His story helped me to strategize and organize a game plan to get my health back under control. He is my inspiration and the one person I know who can truly relate to my COVID-19 experience.

INTRODUCTION

If you look up the words "unprecedented times" in the dictionary, undoubtedly you will see somewhere in the search results words such as "2020" and "pain". The untimely and tragic killings of both George Floyd and Breonna Taylor, and others, reminded African Americans that systematic and individual racism continues to thrive in our nation. Then, the long awaited 2020 Presidential Election. Personally, I had been counting the days until the 2020 election since the 2016 election.

I was excited to see former Vice President Joe Biden, a Democrat who served as vice president under President Barack Obama, squaring off against the Republican Incumbent, President Donald J. Trump, for the nation's top political office. Even after the American people had spoken, and elected Joe Biden as the President Elect by more than six million votes, President Trump still attempted to undermine our so-called democratic process, and disenfranchise voters. Specifically, those who, instead of going to the polls on election day, opted to stay safe and either vote early, or vote by mail. Since he lost the election, no one was really surprised by what he did next—refusing to concede and allow vital government departments to assist the transition team assembled by President Elect Joe Biden.

Together with Vice President Elect Kamala Harris, the nation's first woman and first woman of color to be elected as vice president, Trump's attempts curtailed any preparations to tackle what may be the biggest obstacle of any incoming administration. A problem that Donald Trump refused to acknowledge as a global issue both before the election, and after[1]. Then, there was the global pandemic known as the coronavirus (COVID-19) that ravaged the world. Without any known cure, millions of American lives have been impacted, and thousands have died. As I write this book, vaccines are being produced—but far too late, in my opinion.

My name is Marques Andre Eason, Esq., and this is my COVID-19 story. I am one of over a million Americans that were infected by the coronavirus[2]. Ultimately, my life was spared by the grace of GOD, but it certainly was touch and go. Someone else could be telling my story posthumously. But, instead, here I am sharing my personal survival story. After engaging in the biggest battle of my life. It goes without saying that I am overwhelmingly fortunate and blessed to still be here, with a voice to testify proudly that I am a living witness to GOD's miracles. The scripture tells us that we wrestle not against flesh and blood, but against the powers of this dark world and the spiritual forces of evil in the heavenly realms.[3] In short, the devil came for me, and tried

---

1   He continues to do so even as I write this book.
2   A figure that continues to rise every day as I write this book.
3   Ephesians 6:12

his best to take me out. But what the devil did not realize was that the power of prayer is real, and I had GOD, and a nation of prayer warriors that were not going to let me die without a fight.

I Ain't Done Living Yet is my story about how I recovered from COVID-19 by the grace of GOD. I went to hell and back and survived. Initially, I refused to call it COVID-19 because I thought it was just the media's shorthand way of describing the clinical term, coronavirus. Later, a friend of mine, Vince McCant, who also caught the virus, educated me on why it is called COVID-19. Vince told me that coronavirus had been around for some time, and that this strand of the coronavirus is called COVID-19. Never could I have imagined that I would go through so much and live to tell this story.

I caught the virus during its initial wave in the U.S., specifically in the State of Illinois. Government officials could only react to the onset of the pandemic by issuing mandatory stay-at-home orders, mask mandates, and banning indoor dining at sit-down restaurants. This was all in an effort to curb the spread of the virus that had no known cure, treatment, or available vaccine. During this first wave, doctors around the world shared information and research as initial treatments were on a trial and error basis. All of this was prior to Operation WARP SPEED—the one good thing that President Trump did while in office. This U.S. government initiative facilitated and accelerated the development, manufacturing, and distribution of COVID-19 vaccines in the U.S.—producing a much-needed solution in record breaking time[4].

I spent 40 days in the hospital fighting several significant life-threatening battles brought on by the effects of COVID-19. I have recovered for the most part, but I will never be the same again. When I was seventeen, I got robbed at gunpoint while on a college tour visiting friends at their apartment complex in East Point, Atlanta, Georgia. I thought that was the closest I would ever come to death. But, my ordeal with the coronavirus was scarier, and much closer to death, than looking into a gun barrel. I owe my life to GOD for ensuring that I survived this whole ordeal, and came out on the other side, alive and kicking.

In this memoir, we take an in-depth look into my personal life before, during, and after COVID-19. We will explore my teenage years and the challenges my family faced during these years; my relationships and financial challenges as an adult; bouts with depression and homelessness; and the defining moments that molded me into the man that I am today. Hopefully, this memoir will provide insight into the seven years of frustration I endured before finally, and triumphantly, passing the Illinois Bar exam and being sworn in as an attorney. Finally, we will take a closer look at the health challenges I had before COVID-19, and the battle for my life

---

4 "Fact Sheet: Explaining Operation Warp Speed". US Department of Health and Human Services. November 10, 2020. Retrieved November 24, 2020.

that ensued while infected with COVID-19 (to the extent that I remember). This book will also explore how GOD's mercy and grace spared my life, and how a second chance at life continues to serve as an example of GOD's testimony.

Additionally, I would like to use this memoir to shine a light on the family and friends who played a significant role in this whole ordeal. I genuinely believe that having a strong support system while battling the coronavirus is critical to surviving it. But overall, I pray that my story and the daily journals that were kept detailing what I went through to overcome the coronavirus, encourages you to see that there is life after the virus. I have a long way to go, and though I may never be completely the same, I am blessed—truly blessed—and can only hope that my story and testimony of survival will inspire anyone who reads it, especially those that may have contracted this deadly virus. You are not alone, and you can thrive after surviving COVID-19.

Not only will this memoir give you clear insights into my life, but it will also help you understand the drive, determination, and perseverance that helped me survive and conquer every challenge I've experienced at each stage of my life. In telling my COVID-19 story, my prayer is that this memoir unlocks doors to my past and shares examples of life challenges that I have faced and overcome, leading up to my battle with the virus. How I've thrived in my day-to-day life, even after dealing with the life-changing and life-threatening events faced as the direct result of my experience with COVID-19, is also a key focus in this book.

PAST

'Your past has given you the strength and the wisdom you have today, so celebrate it. Do not let it haunt you.'

CHAPTER 1

'Difficulties are a setup for GOD to do
something greater. Setbacks are a setup for GOD to
move you towards your destiny'

—Joel Osteen

I was born in LaGrange, Illinois, a southwest suburb of Chicago, on March 10th, 1977. My mother, a public-school teacher, and my father, an engineer, divorced when I was still an infant. After they divorced, my mother moved us to Bolingbrook, IL (a western suburb). I was so young that I have no recollection of the apartment we lived in at the time. Later, we moved to Park Forest South, Illinois (now known as University Park, Illinois) on Marina Court. I went to Montessori school until first grade and Crete Elementary School for second through sixth grade. I spent one year at Crete-Monee Junior High School. In 1991, my mother remarried, and we moved to the south side of Chicago.

Growing up, I was shy. It was hard for me to talk to girls. I was kind of a tweener—not cool enough to be liked by girls, but not geeky enough to be considered a nerd. In grammar school, I got all A's and B's through sixth grade—for the most part. In fifth grade, I got a C+ and the rest were A's. But of course, my mother did not care about the four or five A's I got. All she cared about was why I got that C+. I guess I should have known that being the son of a professional educator, nothing but the best was expected from me. In high school, I became more active in sports, and girls started to notice me more. But, at the same time, my grades slipped significantly. I essentially became a B/C student. Looking back, I realized that I did not try hard enough. At that time, it was more important for me to fit in, rather than being smart.

My dream was to become a professional athlete. At first, I wanted to play football for the Chicago Bears, or become a baseball player for my hometown team: the Chicago White Sox. I had dreams of becoming the star quarterback at each level. When it became clear in high school that I was not cut out for a career in either the National Football League (NFL), or Major League Baseball (MLB), I decided that I wanted to be a computer engineer. In grammar school, I was brilliant in math, but unfortunately, that did not translate into my high school years. So, when I began my journey at the University of Illinois at Urbana-Champaign, my only objective was to pick a major that would lead to financial success.

MY FAMILY/SUPPORT SYSTEM

Despite the obstacles that I faced, like most people, I am truly a derivative of my environment, values, and support system. When you are faced with a life-threatening illness, most times, you tend to reevaluate your priorities and remember the people and life experiences that have pulled you through such dilapidating situations. That is why I am thankful to GOD that He blessed me with so many amazing people—especially my mother Barbara Eason-Watkins. I could not have asked for a better mother.

BARBARA EASON-WATKINS

Born in 1952, and raised on the Southwest Side of Detroit, my mother, Barbara Eason-Watkins was the only child born to my grandparents, Gladys and Ceroy Hollis. She graduated from Cass Technical High School in Detroit and attended the University of Michigan. You have no clue how many times I have had to hear that "Go Blue" chant every time Illinois and Michigan played in a college football game. Of course, Michigan got the best of Illinois most of the time. But every now and then, the "Fighting Illini" surprised us with an incredible season, which often included a victory over the Michigan Wolverines. Those were the years I did not hear that "Go Blue" chant as much. The University of Michigan is also where she met my father.

My mother initially spent her summers working in a Detroit hospital with my uncle John. Uncle John was not my blood uncle. He was my grandparents' neighbor who lived two houses down. She ultimately decided to be a teacher and moved to Chicago. She moved in with my father who was already living there. They got married in 1974, but divorced by 1977 when I was just three months old.

After the divorce, my mother and I moved to an apartment in Bolingbrook, Illinois. I honestly have no memories of living in that place. From there, we moved to what was then Park Forest South (now known as University Park). We lived there until I was 13. My mother married my stepfather, Irv, a life-long practicing dentist, and he moved us back to Chicago—to the home we refer to now as the "Claremont" house. My stepfather and I had a challenging relationship while I was growing up. But the relationship grew stronger in my adult life. He has always supported my mother, especially while I was in the hospital battling COVID-19.

My mother worked for the Chicago Public Schools for 35 years. She started as a primary school teacher at Mahalia Jackson for one year. Then, she spent three years at Scanlon, and six years after that at Carver Primary school. During this time, she earned her master's degree from Chicago State University and began further studies to become a principal. She got the chance to be a principal at Mollison Elementary School on 44th and King Drive, right next to King High School—known for its basketball program back then. She served as principal of Mollison from 1985-1988, before switching to a bigger school, James McCosh Elementary (now called Emmitt Till Elementary), located in the heart of the Woodlawn neighborhood, on 65th and Champlain. She remained at McCosh for 13 years until 2001, when she got a call from then

CEO of Chicago Public Schools (CPS), Arne Duncan. Arne offered her a job in the central office downtown as the Chief Education Officer for Chicago Public Schools. I remember she called me to ask me for my opinion on the offer. She was conflicted about leaving her students at McCosh. I told her that this was a golden opportunity where she could make a difference for more kids, and not just limit herself to those at McCosh. She accepted the job and held it for nearly 10 years.

In 2009, following the historic Presidential Election, Arne resigned from CPS after being nominated as the U.S. Secretary of Education by President Barack Obama. My mother was offered the opportunity to go with him, but did not want to travel back and forth between Washington D.C and Chicago. I was very disappointed that she did not take the job. I would have loved to have had a home in the D.C. area. In 2009, I remember reading a Chicago Sun-Times article that had pegged my mother as the favorite to replace Arne as Chief Executive Officer of CPS. However, the mayor overlooked her and appointed Ron Huberman, a former police officer, to the position. She never said much about it, but I knew my mother was disappointed and felt unappreciated after all she had done for CPS. In late 2010, she progressed and became the superintendent of the Michigan City Area Schools district. Ironically, the school district office is right down the street from the home she and my stepfather bought in Michigan City. She has been there ever since and remains happy and fulfilled.

GLADYS AND CEROY HOLLIS
(MATERNAL GRANDPARENTS)

Outside of my mother's care, my grandparents played an instrumental role in my life as well. My grandfather, Ceroy, worked for Chrysler for over forty years before he retired. He died from a blood clot in his leg when I was 13 in 1990, the day before Valentine's Day. Before he died, my grandparents purchased adjacent burial spots in a mausoleum in Detroit. My grandmother, Gladys, was a teacher for forty years before she retired. She was amazing, caring and loved me to death. She helped my mother pay for my university tuition, so I had no financial aid debt when I graduated from undergrad. She also helped me pay for my brand-new Ford Explorer in 2002. My grandmother was a GOD-fearing praying woman. I know she always prayed. She died of cancer in February 2008, almost to the day that my grandfather died seventeen years earlier (1991). Before she died, I went home for Christmas and we visited her at the University of Chicago hospital, the same hospital where I engaged in my battle with COVID-19. I knew that my visit would probably be the last time I would see her alive. In a private moment with her, I apologized for being such a "difficult" grandson and thanked her for everything she had done for me. I was happy to at least have had the opportunity to say goodbye to her before she died—something that I did not get a chance to do with my grandfather because he died so suddenly. Even in death, she left me thirty-one thousand dollars in U.S. bonds—money that I foolishly squandered away in less than six months.

LARAS EDRED EASON

I have always idolized my father. Laras Edred Eason was born in Birmingham, Alabama in 1950, and was the second of five siblings born to Louise and Amos Eason Sr, my paternal grandparents. My grandfather eventually moved the family to Pontiac, Michigan, and he too, just like my mother's father, worked in the automotive industry, General Motors, for forty years. My grandfather died of lymphoma in 1995, when I was 18. My grandmother is a retired nurse and is still with us today—she is in her 90s, but moves around like she is in her forties. My father's parents had five children—Amos Jr, my oldest uncle, my father, aunt Cynthia (or Rita), uncle Daryl, and aunt Angela. Angela is my favorite aunt—partially because we are only 11 years apart. She would babysit my sisters and I during the summers that I spent in Pontiac. My aunt Cynthia is Sabrina's mother—my favorite cousin. In 2015, when I was preparing to go to law school, Cynthia told me that "GOD has a different plan for you," and regarding my dreams of becoming a lawyer, she told me: "that ship has sailed." I am sure she meant well, but her words still affect me to this day—my mother or father also did not approve of what she said. In fact, her comments were a major motivating factor that pushed me to finally sit and pass the bar in

February 2017. If nothing else, I was motivated and determined to prove her wrong.

I was the only child from my parent's marriage, but my father went on to have other children. After he and my mother divorced, my father moved back to Pontiac where he met my stepmother, Lorine. In 1980, my sister, Stesha, was born. For the longest time, it was just us during the summers. In 1984, Lorine and my father got married. In 1985, my baby sister, Erica, was born. Erica and I are eight years apart, but growing up, we became the closest of siblings.

My father was my biggest supporter when I became an adult. My mother was everything to me during my childhood years, but my dad stepped up significantly as I got older and needed advice. He was not judgmental and gave advice without insisting on the financial consequences of my decisions. My mother, understandably, was the educator and was always concerned about me making decisions and taking part in things that put money in my pocket. She was adamant about getting involved with people who could bring something to the table i.e., money—not just benefitting from my status or hard-earned money.

During the summers, my dad made it to all my baseball games, and always preached about GOD as I was growing up. He was not the perfect father, and had his faults—but he was "my father", and perfect for me. Lord knows his faith was battle-tested on this one—his only son, lying in a hospital bed, barely clinging to life. Tested, but never wavered.

MY DAUGHTERS

I have two children of my own, Amber, my oldest, and Vivian. Amber was born on November 4th, 1994, and Vivian was born on March 16th, 1995 (six days after my birthday). Amber, the oldest of my two girls, was born six months earlier than Vivian. I love both of my daughters equally, but when Amber came into my life, she was truly the best thing that ever happened to me. Amber is mature beyond her years. At a very young age, she has mastered the art of kindness and treats everyone she encounters with politeness and respect. She is smart, extremely talented, and humble. Most importantly, she loves GOD and puts GOD first in everything she does.

Amber has always been a superstar in the making. When she was in high school, Karen, her mother, would take her to the studio on the weekends to record music—all weekend—with her girl group. Again, Amber has always been a very humble young woman. But Karen and I knew it was just a matter of time before she would be ready to step out on her own as a performing artist.

Amber won her first talent show at Webb Bridge Middle School in Atlanta, performing "If I Ain't Got You" by one of her idols, Alicia Keys. Her mother and maternal grandparents did an excellent job of keeping her grounded, and getting her involved in church, so performing on stage became natural to her once she reached adulthood. As the years went by, Amber started performing solo. I set up several shows for her to perform, and arranged for vocal lessons with my friend Keisha Jackson—daughter of soul legend Mille Jackson. Keisha is a great teacher, and really pushes her students. But for some reason, while their overall relationship was good, things just did not work out. Eventually, I paired her up with Ametria Dock, another vocal coach based in Atlanta. With Ametria, it was like a light bulb switched on. Amber really felt comfortable with Ametria, and the chemistry was great between them.

Amber was on the cusp of launching her music career, with me as her manager. In 2019, she decided to change her stage name from "Amber Makayla" to "Sauvi DuVin". At first, I was concerned about the name change, but I began to like it as time went on. Sauvi is a superstar in the making and had just performed in Chicago for me at my birthday party—where I believe I actually caught the coronavirus[5]. Currently, she has a song on iTunes called "Luv For You", and several more in the making. She has opened for the likes of Maze featuring Frankie Beverly and the Isley Brothers at the Verizon Theater at Grand Prairie, while performing with an Atlanta based concert band known as "The City." She was scheduled to open for the Whispers and Maze in Atlanta. However, due to the production truck being late, and the neighborhood, where the venue was located, having a sound ordinance, they were cut from the show.

---

5   It is also possible that I caught the virus at a local pub in my old Beverly neighborhood.

I used to promote live music shows in Atlanta under the guise of "Marques Eason Entertainment". Nowadays, I just promote Sauvi DuVin shows and act as her manager. The future for Sauvi DuVin was extremely bright, and we were looking forward to the possibilities to further her career in 2020. However, the pandemic came down like the black plague, and all our 2020 plans for Sauvi DuVin came to a screeching halt.

In addition to her music career, Amber graduated from Georgia State University in 2018 with a bachelor's degree in Political Science. Initially, she had to withdraw for financial reasons, but was determined to go back and finish what she started—and she did. Amber was one of the reasons why I needed to pass the bar exam. Initially, I did not realize that she was observing my every move. Once I did, I wanted her to see me finish what I started, in the hopes of motivating her to do the same. To this day, Karen and I are still great friends. The three of us are a remarkably close family unit. My relationship with Amber is great.

With Vivian, however, not so much, but it was not always like that. Unlike my relationship with Karen, Vivian's mother, Rhonda, and I do not have the same friendly relationship. When Vivian was younger, we had a great relationship until she turned fourteen. Amongst other things, her mother has been angry at me for years, and filled Vivian's head with untrue stories. But I think the biggest thing that made our relationship go south was that, while I was living in Atlanta,

I started developing a closer relationship with Amber. I think Vivian felt slighted because she felt like I did not give her the same attention that she used to get when I lived in Chicago. I guess I can understand her feeling that way. That, coupled with her mother being in her ear, might have convinced Vivian that I do not love her like I love Amber. The truth is, and always has been, that I love both of them the same. Vivian has said a lot of hurtful things over the years, but she's still my daughter. For now, I have left the door open for her to come back and rebuild our relationship when she is ready.

OTHA SMITH JR.

One of my best friends, Otha, whom his friends called "O," was more like an older brother to Kris and I than a friend. He named Kris, my brother, "Ghost," in honor of Omar Hardwick's character on the TV show *Power* because when it was time for us to hang out, Kris would always disappear. He would take so long to meet us at our agreed spot, and otherwise, could not be found.

At any rate, O was from the South Side of Chicago (62nd at Saint Lawrence). O attended middle school at the University of Chicago Lab School, Hales Franciscan high school on 49th and Cottage Grove, and the University of Illinois at Urbana-Champaign for college—where he crossed paths with Kris and I. O was two years older than us, and he, along with our friend April, were the founders of this hangout group that will forever be known as CREW. Kris and I became part of CREW once we arrived on campus.

O loved his friends and was a HUGE baseball fan. If you know Chicago, then you know that the city is divided when it comes to baseball. If you were from the South Side, you were a Chicago White Sox fan. If you were from the North Side, you were a Chicago Cubs fan. But that was not the case with O. Despite being born and raised on the South Side, O was a huge Cubs fan. Mainly because when we were younger, cable was too expensive, and most of us only had local channels on the TV. The White Sox played most of their games on Sports Vision—now Fox Sports. Meanwhile, the Cubs played all their games on Chicago's local station, Channel 9 or WGN. O became a fan since he only had access to Cubs' games. We used to tease O for years about how bad the Chicago Cubs were—especially when we were introduced to Facebook in 2006.

Otha Smith Jr. passed away in his sleep at the age of 43. The coroner later determined that O passed away in the early morning, between 3 am and 5 am, and that he died of congestive heart failure. Over 10 years ago, while in Vegas, O became sick and had to be hospitalized. He was diagnosed with Kidney Renal Failure and had to have dialysis sessions for the next several years. In 2014, O had a kidney transplant and was removed from dialysis. In the months before his death, he had mentioned that his other kidney that had not been replaced was beginning to affect his new kidney and doctors were changing his medication. We had even seen pictures of him on his Facebook page, working out regularly. All signs pointed to him getting better and healthier. His death hit us all like a Mack truck that came out of nowhere, especially me. I had a difficult time accepting that O was gone.

Soon after he died, I was in a panic about my own health. Though I did not have health insurance at the time, I made sure to get a physical that year. I was forty-one. But in March 2020, as it became apparent that something was wrong with my health, thinking about the fact that O was forty-three years old when he died, was heavy on my mind. I began to wonder if I would succumb to the same fate and pass away just after celebrating my forty-third birthday. Nevertheless, GOD had other plans for me, and for that, I am so grateful.

THE TRANSITION

My journey at the University of Illinois had its own challeng-es. During my senior year in high school, I learned that I was about to be a father to my daughter Vivian. Additionally, with just a few weeks left in the semester, my stepfather had kicked me out of the house with good reason. I had done a long list of things, including taking my mother's car from the garage, and going to see a girlfriend whose mother worked nights, and ultimately, for taking Irv's gun, an heirloom that I did not know at the time was left to him by his own father. The night I was kicked out, I called my guys, Donald Dennis and Gerald Holden, who were already at the University of Illinois, to let them know that I was headed to Champaign that night. I ran to the 103rd Street bus stop, and took a bus to the 95th Street Dan Ryan Station, where I jumped on a train headed towards downtown Chicago. I got off at the Roosevelt stop and walked towards the Greyhound Bus Station so that I could head down to the University of Illinois at Urbana-Champaign.

Along the way, as I walked to the Greyhound Station to buy a bus ticket to Champaign, Illinois, I stopped on the bridge just above the Chicago River to throw away Irv's gun that I had taken before I left the house. I had taken it mainly to protect myself because of some shit I got myself into that year. However, it represented everything that I was not, so I had to let it go.

While I was in Champaign, I reached out to Ron Woolfolk and Pamela Greer, the directors of the transition program I had registered to attend in the Fall. Ron and Pam were also a part of "Bridge" as well, the summer component of the transition program. This summer Bridge component required you to complete six weeks of intensive college-level course work during the summer, while residing in the university residence halls. You had to get a "C" or better to be admitted into the University. When I met with both Ron and Pam, I explained everything that had happened, including the fact that I had just become a father and needed to be home during the summer. However, I reiterated that I was still committed to being part of the program.

Nonetheless, after the drama surrounding Vivian's birth, my priorities changed slightly, and I just wanted to spend time with my daughter. At that time, I did not know that I had another older daughter Amber. But that is another story in and of itself. Because of my new obligations, I intended to get into the transition program in the Fall, but not Bridge. I hoped that I could spend the summer in Chicago with my newborn daughter, continue working as a short order cook at Janson's Drive-In, and leave in August 1995 for University. But clearly GOD had a different plan for me then. I ended up quitting my job as a short order cook before graduating and moving to Champaign a few months earlier than I expected to start the Bridge program. This was probably the first time I learned that GOD always knows what is best for you, even if it's not what you want to do. Thy will be done.

Dr. Luke Helm, my family therapist at the time, was my whisperer. He understood things about me at age seventeen and eighteen, that I did not understand myself. He understood everything I said and could easily explain my madness to me, and those that did not understand me. Dr. Helm also had a relationship with Ron and Pam of the Bridge/Transition Program. Not only was he a former graduate of the University of Illinois, but his children were alumni as well, so he was familiar with the institution. At any rate—unbeknownst to me, and with my mother's blessing—Dr. Helm had orchestrated the arrangement with Ron and Pam for me to attend Bridge during the summer. That was the exact opposite of what I wanted to do. All I could think of at the time was that

I needed to stay in Chicago for Vivian. I had not seen her since the first week she was born, and I figured that if I left for Champaign in June, I might never see her again. But Ron, Pam, Dr. Helm, and my mother, all convinced me that if I did not go to school, I could not fulfill my fatherly duties and provide the best for her. I was left with no choice. Despite my reservations, it was clear that my journey into the University of Illinois would begin in June 1995 as a summer Bridge program student.

MY MAD MAN STORY

I remember it like it was yesterday—June 23rd, 1995. I boarded the bus that picked us up at UIC on Halsted Street in Chicago and headed south down Interstate 57 (I-57) to Illinois Street Residence Hall (ISR) on the University of Illinois campus in Urbana. There was no star in the sky that I missed during the first three or four weeks of the six-week program. I was physically present, but my mind was back in Chicago, clouded with thoughts of Vivian, and the mess I had left at home with my mother and stepfather. I was surviving Bridge, I was not failing any classes, and it seemed like I would make the grades I needed to pass Bridge. Nevertheless, Ron and Pam had spoken to me several times to encourage me to refocus, but nothing seemed to work.

During the fourth week of the program, they sat down with a group of students, handing out progress reports. They got down to the last two, which ended up being me, and this guy named Carlos. Unlike me, Carlos was failing every class. Yet, they sent us both home for the weekend to evaluate whether we genuinely wanted to be in the Bridge program and at the University. I remember what Ron said like it was yesterday: 'We've come as far as we can go with you two. It's up to you to decide if you truly want to be here.' I was angry and confused. Why did they have me sitting in this room next to a guy who was failing, even though I was doing okay in my classes? Eventually, I did the only thing that I knew how to do—I went to the computer lab and began to write.

I started with quotes from Batman, MC Hammer, and James Brown. The quotes were 'I am the terror that walks in the night' and 'too legit to quit'. This was just the intro to the story I began to write. I called it: *"The Mad Man Stories."* *The Mad Man stories* were about a fearless young man, with "mojo". One day, that fearlessness and mojo had disappeared. He searched high and low for this "mojo", but could not find it. But at last, he seemed to find the path back to his inner confident self. This inner confident self was located at *10401 South Claremont*—my home in Chicago. I cried the whole time I was writing this story. Pam was in the computer lab with us at the time. I printed out two copies of the story, handed a copy to her, and went back upstairs to my room in ISR.

The next day, I learned that Ron and Pam had distributed the story to all the other tutor counselors working in the program, all of whom had read it. Ron had also sent the story to Dr. Helm. I remember thinking "oh sh*t, what have

I done?" I did not know how Dr. Helm was going to react. Would he think I embarrassed him because he vouched for me to be in the program? All the program staff and administrators thought I was crazy because they did not understand the story. Would Dr. Helm think I was crazy as well? Hell, I, myself, did not understand the story. No one had a clue as to what I was talking about—except Dr. Helm.

Upon returning home to Chicago, Dr. Helm had scheduled a meeting between my mother, my stepfather, and myself. I learned about this the day before, and I was ready to leave Chicago at that moment. During the meeting, that urgency to leave heightened when the first words out of my stepfather's mouth were, "You need me". I was ready to go instantly, and almost got up and walked out. I felt the meeting would be pointless and was just an opportunity for Irv to continue what I felt were his berated threats. But I was not afraid of him anymore. It had been four months since the night I was kicked out of the house. I found a way to survive all this time leading up to that day, and I found a way to survive moving forward, with or without him. But I knew that it was my mother, more than me, that needed peace and resolution. And looking back, I know that Irv felt the same way. Throughout the meeting, my mother was in tears, and it was just an all-around mess. Dr. Helm always described my mother as the "meat between two pieces of bread".

As time went on, the conversation was going nowhere. I tried to leave the office. I had enough money to get on public transportation, head downtown, buy myself a Greyhound ticket and go back to Champaign. I had seen enough. I knew what I had to do in Bridge. I was ready to show Ron and Pam that I was willing to do whatever just to not have to come back to Chicago. I even thought that being homeless was better than dealing with this situation. But before I could leave, Dr. Helm asked me to wait, and trust him. All I could do was pause. I was not sure what to do. After all, Dr. Helm was the only person that I trusted at that time. More importantly, I knew that he had never let me down in the past, and whatever he was trying to accomplish, I was sure that he would not let me down now. So, I decided to stay and sat back down in my seat in his office.

Dr. Helm began reading the story to my mother and stepfather, and this made me upset. I immediately asked him, "What are you doing?" He responded, "Marques, I'm asking you to trust me!" I sat quietly and let him finish reading. I was sure my stepfather already thought I was crazy. He thought I was a thug or hoodlum because I wore my hat to the back. He did not really know me at the time, but I did not want him to hear my story, which still did not make sense to me either. I did not want him to add crazy to his list. But I knew that Dr. Helm had a good reason for sharing with them what I had written, so as difficult as this was, I had to trust him. Besides, Dr. Helm was the only person in the room that knew what I was trying to say.

This "inner mad man" was at 10401 South Claremont, he continued. Dr. Helm explained to my mother that I was trying to express that I was ready to come home. I could not believe it and was in complete awe. Dr. Helm's explanation was starting to make sense even before he finished. He could see through my story that I was crying out for help. That I was trying to tell anyone who would listen that I was ready to go home and face my biggest fear at the time—my stepfather. In my mind, I was not afraid of him anymore. I just wanted to take back control of my own life and move on. But I could never do that with this "dark cloud" hovering over my head. I had to face him.

Subconsciously, I knew that it was the only way to break free and move on with my life, starting afresh at the University of Illinois. Eventually, I finally had a chance to say my peace. That I just wanted to be left alone and knew that if I wanted to, I could break their marriage. But I had no desire to do so. I just wanted out—to be free, and to be left alone. My mother tried so hard to make us a family, but I did not want that at the time. I had a father. He was not the greatest, but he was my dad, and he was active in my life the best way he knew how. I had accepted that my mother decided to spend the rest of her life with Irv. But that was her decision, I did not marry him. I just wanted out so that I could move on with my life. Apparently, that resonated loud and clear throughout the room that day, and I believe that my point was made.

I was now ready to head back and finish the Bridge program with a bang and start my studies at the University of Illinois. I returned that weekend feeling like a new man, with a renewed purpose. I also remember feeling like this session had brought me peace of mind as it related to my younger daughter Vivian as well. Somehow, I knew I could not do anything at that time, but I never forgot about her. I knew the perfect moment would present itself when I could see her again and be ready to fight for her. But for now, I knew I had to focus and get myself together. I knew the only place for me to do that was at the University of Illinois. But more importantly, I knew that there was no way in hell I would go back home to face my stepfather as a failure ever again. I had accomplished what I needed to accomplish. I had faced my fear of going back home. I said what I needed to say for me to move on with my life, and start a fresh at the University of Illinois.

Dr. Helm died of a heart attack about 14 years ago on September 5th, 2006. I loved that man as if he were my own father, and he clearly loved me as if I was his own son. To this day, I hate myself for not keeping in touch with him, or if nothing else, making sure he knew that I loved him, how much he meant to me, how much I appreciated everything he did for me, and everything he was to me at a time when I clearly needed him the most.

After this whole debacle, I had a different perspective of my stepfather. He has played a major role in my mother's, and

Vivian's life. I realized that I was no saint growing up. Even though my stepfather had been a part of my life since I was two or three years old, I am sure it was difficult trying to raise a child that was not his own. But he did the best he could. No, he was not perfect. But neither was I. As we have progressed through life, he has played a major role in supporting my business ventures. My stepfather was a dentist. He ran a successful dental practice for 47 years before retiring in September 2020 and had several successful real estate investment ventures as well. He is the reason I knew I was making the right decision to pursue my entrepreneurial interests. Irv always taught me that in corporate America, you could only progress so much. But when it came to being an entrepreneur, he always said that there was no ceiling for success.

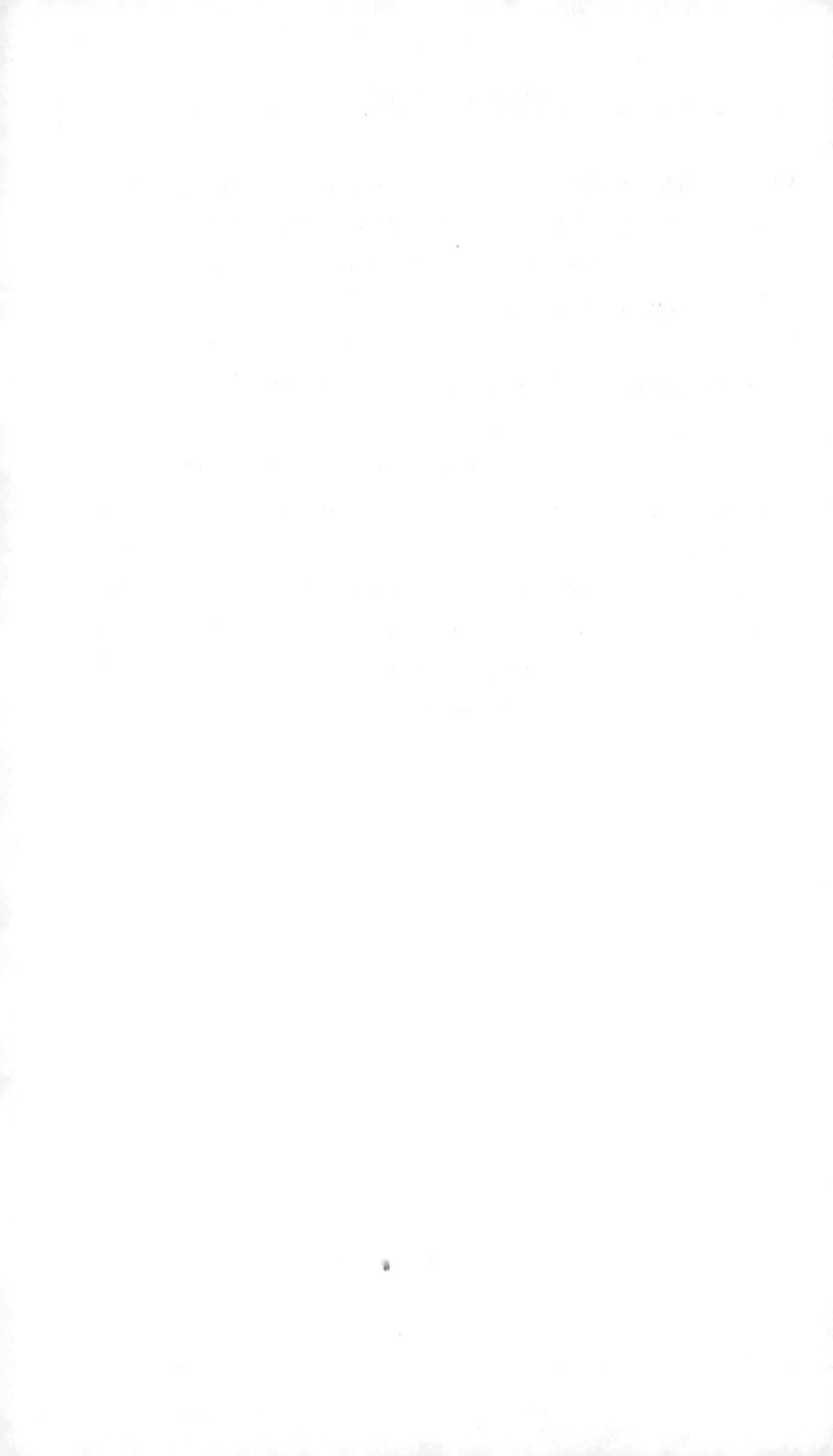

CHAPTER 2

'The ultimate measure of a man is not where he stands in moments of convenience and comfort, but where he stands at times of challenge and controversy'

—Dr. King.

My first semester at the University of Illinois was a continuance of the last two weeks of Bridge. I was ready, but I still had to prove myself. I did not want to be the average student that I was in high school. I could not take a math major, but the task now was finding something that was the best fit for me. Most people around me suggested law school, but I did not want to do a "pre-law major" for the next four years. I wanted to do something that I would enjoy and get excited about learning in the next four years. I spent several days meeting with my academic advisor, Kristian, exploring different majors. Kristian recommended that I speak to department heads before ultimately deciding on a major. Even though I went through the first semester at U of I undeclared, I ended the semester with a 3.0 GPA.

Ron and Pam called Dr. Helm first, who then called my stepfather and gave him the news. Irv then told my mother and me. Looking back, I think Dr. Helm intentionally told my stepfather first on purpose. When Irv told me about my grades, he seemed shocked that I was not surprised or in awe by my first semester grades. I had been tracking my grades all through the Christmas break. That said, all I could think about was what he told me that night while he was kicking me out of the house: 'When you get to Champaign, those white boys will kick your ass.' If anything, I felt vindicated. I later heard him say that he had friends whose children went to U of I and did not survive their first semester. But I knew I was not done. Nothing short of graduating from U of I was acceptable to me.

During the Spring semester of 1996, I was still searching for a major, and then it happened. By mistake, or in passing, Kristian mentioned something about Sports Management and Leisure Studies. Immediately, I began doing my research on what the University of Illinois offered. Then, I learned that the Sports Management program was housed in the College of Applied Life Studies, in the Department of Leisure Studies—now known as "Recreation, Sport, and Tourism". At the time, there were not that many black students in that Department, but that was common given that out of thirty-six thousand students at U of I, only two thousand were African American. I ended up registering for Leisure Studies 100, the introductory course, with one of my best friends, Abdullah ("Dullah"). Dullah originally wanted to study Event Planning or Hotel Tourism Management. Today, he is a veteran Chicago Police Officer—go figure.

I took five classes during the Spring 1996 Semester. I earned all A's and one B and earned a 3.7 GPA. My favorite class that semester was my Rhetoric 102 class, led by writing instructor, Syd Slobodnik. Syd was one of the writing instructors during Bridge in that summer. I did not have Syd during Bridge, but his reputation preceded him. Syd also had a reputation for being a hard grader, and he rarely awarded A's. I was late for my first meeting with him, and Syd ripped me a new one. I had also missed three classes in the first two weeks—the class met on Tuesdays and Thursdays with our one-on-one sessions on Fridays. He warned me that I would fail the course if I did not get my act together.

Naturally, that pissed me off. But he was right. Though I was slacking, I was determined to change his impression of me by the end of the semester. I ended up getting an A minus on the first paper I wrote for his class. I told Ron, Pam, and Kristian, and they were surprised because, as they all said, "Syd doesn't give A's". Little did they know, I had already decided that I would be the first person, in a long time, to get an A in his course. Every week after that, I would write my paper in advance of the deadline, and schedule office hours with him to talk about how I could make my writing better. Syd would give me feedback, and I would make the improvements before the final submission deadlines for each assignment. I got an A every time after that, and an A in his course. That was the first time I really knew that I could write.

That following summer, I stayed in Champaign and worked as a Bridge tutor/counselor. No one my age had ever done that before. The program usually only hired tutors and counselors after their sophomore year, or later. But Ron and Pam took a chance on me after seeing how passionate I was about the program. It was a challenge to say the least. It was hard being on the other side, tutor counselor versus a student, but I eventually got through Bridge that year. In my remaining years at U of I, I served as a writing tutor for the program—mainly under Syd Slobodnik for the Summer Bridge Program. Dullah and I also spent our summers as participants in the Summer Research Opportunities Program (SROP) where we completed research topics related to Leisure Studies, Sports Management, and Event Management. We both graduated from U of I in May 1999, and I relocated to Atlanta, Georgia, to work as a Baseball Operations Intern for the Atlanta Braves.

In Atlanta, I got the opportunity to work alongside John Schuerholz, the Atlanta Braves General Manager. Mr. Schuerholz was the brains behind the Atlanta Braves' championship run in the 1990s. I had the chance to see how things operated behind the scenes on a day-to-day basis, and witnessed the activities involved in strategizing and developing a major league roster. But I was a horrible, *horrible* intern. Although the experience was good, I learned many hard lessons about hard work and commitment, and what can happen in that kind of environment when you do not put your best foot forward, or keep your mouth shut. After the summer internship with the Braves, I returned to Chicago.

When I returned to Chicago, I moved back to live with my mother and stepfather for a year. I worked as a temp for a staffing company on various accounting assignments. Eventually, I got a job with the Chicago Park District's Lakefront Region as a Human Resources Coordinator. Our main office was housed inside the South Shore Cultural Center. I was the HR Coordinator for the entire lakefront region. I was responsible for staffing all the seasonal laborers, instructors, and other staff members for the Lakefront Region of the Park District as well. I was making only twenty-five thousand dollars per year, but I could pay my bills and pay my parents' rent—three hundred fifty dollars per month.

In the Spring of 2000, I took another shot at professional sports, and accepted a Public Relations Internship with the Chicago White Sox. I was only being paid one thousand one hundred dollars per month. But at the time, it was worth the shot of getting a second chance at working for a Major league baseball organization—especially my beloved hometown team, the Chicago White Sox. That year, the White Sox finished the regular season in first place in the American League Central Division, but were eliminated in the first round of the playoffs. Overall, the experience was better, but the outcome was the same. I realized I could not hack it as an intern. I was starting to see a pattern develop in my professional career. It seemed like I was finding it extremely hard working for people—I did not like it and knew there had to be something better.

A NEW DIRECTION

After leaving the White Sox baseball organization, I worked briefly as an Admissions Counselor with the Illinois Institute of Technology (IIT). I stayed there for five months before deciding to move back to Atlanta in the Spring of 2001. I had interviewed with several companies but had not secured a job in Atlanta until I moved. When I arrived, I finally received an offer from Coca-Cola Enterprises (CCE) as a Help Desk Analyst. I had always been good with computers and technology—something I had picked up from my dad and godfather. I began working for CCE in March 2001. I stayed at CCE for four years, relocating to Los Angeles in 2002 after being promoted to a Field Technician position. In 2003, I relocated to Tampa, after being promoted again to a lead position at their Shared Services Facility in Tampa (Brandon), Florida. Los Angeles was the only place where I honestly enjoyed being an employee. To this day, the best manager I ever worked for was Farzin Samadani.

Farzin was born in Iran, but when you heard him speak, he was a New Yorker through and through. Like me, he had been promoted to IT Manager and relocated to Los Angeles from Columbia, Maryland. Our team was very diverse. Like Farzin, there was Ronald Raghoo, who was from Trinidad, and had migrated from New York. Marty Horecky was the

Senior Field IT Analyst and was from Boston. There was also Hai Do, who was Vietnamese and the sole remaining member of the previous Field IT team in the Los Angeles office. Robin Mullins was our mobile computing specialist, who worked out of the facility in Rancho Cucamonga, and Donna DeSousa was our voice technology liaison and based in San Diego. Finally, I cannot forget Steve Ramaker who was the true heart and soul of our team and the one who had been there the longest. When we arrived, he technically was not part of the Field IT team at the time. But shortly thereafter, Farzin welcomed him into the fold, and we made sure that he felt like he was part of our family.

During my time in L.A., I was fond of using the word "WOOSA", a famous phrase from the movie *Bad Boys II*, which premiered in early 2003. Our Field IT team had a lot of issues to address across all the facilities in South California— as far north as Santa Maria and as far south as San Diego. It was not easy. The business customers we supported did not trust us at first. The previous team had screwed them over on several occasions, so we had to work hard to earn their trust back. It took a lot of patience, and a lot of *WOOSA's*. But as a unit, we accomplished everything we set out to achieve. Consequently, Raghoo and I shared a similar mantra from the movie—*'we ride together, we die together. Bad boys for life.'*

Farzin was the best manager that I ever worked for. In many ways, he was like Phil Jackson, who led the Bulls and Lakers to 13 NBA Championships collectively. We each had different personalities, and he managed each of us fairly, but differently. Farzin gave me the space to be who I needed to be. We had our moments, where he had to correct me as my supervisor just like everyone else. But to this day, he is the only manager I could ever work for.

In the Fall of 2004, I was visiting San Diego for work when I met up with my Uncle Daryl (Eason) at the bar of the hotel I was staying at. At the time, he lived in San Diego with his wife and two kids. This was undoubtedly one of the absolute best times of my life. It was the first time I truly got to hang out with my uncle, as an adult. And boy did we let loose. We discussed many things that night, including how happy and content I was working for CCE, how much I loved going to work every day, how I looked forward to achieving work tasks, and hated going home at night. At the time, I still had a girlfriend in Atlanta, Kiya, who I was missing dearly. She could not handle the stresses of a long-distance relationship and started seeing someone else. If I was busy at work, I would not have the time to think about our relationship. But when I got home, that is all I thought about—the two of them together. It burned me up inside. But outside of that, I finally found a place where I belonged—with my co-workers.

Daryl understood the highs and lows of how I was feeling. He said that all the success I was experiencing while working in corporate America was great, but he felt that I was shortchanging myself and that I needed to consider pursuing my dreams of going to law school. I was not necessarily surprised by the comment itself. I was just surprised that it came from him. There we were, the two of us in our drunken stupor, discussing my future as an attorney. Like I said, it was a fun night. But he planted the seed in my head that I needed to transition to something that I had been wanting and planning to do after college. Corporate America had become a comfort to me and had postponed what I really wanted to do. I had not forgotten about law school—I just put it to the side for the time being.

So, I decided it was time for me to leave Coca-Cola Enterprises, heed my Uncle Daryl's advice, and pursue law school. Unfortunately, I did not start applying to law school until March 2005, which was very late to apply for the Fall 2005 semester. I applied to over fifty law schools and got rejected fifty times. At the time, my LSAT score was considerably low by law school standards. So, I hired a private tutor, David Hammer, who was a Tampa native, to help me prepare for the October 2005 administration of the LSAT. I raised my score to what was more acceptable to law schools at the time. Then, I started applying to law schools for the Fall 2006 semester admission.

Since my plans to go to law school were placed on hold, I decided to accept an offer with Deloitte Services LP ("Deloitte") as a Technical Support Analyst. They offered me my choice of locations: Atlanta, Georgia, Washington D.C., or Charlotte, NC. In hindsight, I probably should have chosen Atlanta. But I wanted to try something new considering that

I had spent so much time in Atlanta before—I knew I could always come back. Washington D.C. was too expensive for an annual salary of fifty thousand dollars. Therefore, I decided to relocate where my favorite cousin Sabrina lived—Charlotte, North Carolina.

I started work in Charlotte in January 2006 and moved in with Sabrina. Things were not as rosy as I expected. We were just two different people. Even though we loved each other immensely, we just could not live together. Things got so bad, that I moved out and stayed in a friend's guest bedroom—a woman I was dating at the time—while I looked for my own place. After just three days, I found an apartment in the University area of Charlotte.

On April 3rd, 2006, the day after signing my lease and moving into the apartment, I went to my post office box in Downtown Charlotte, just down the street from the Deloitte office. I had my mail forwarded from my address in Tampa to that post office box. At the time, I had applied to sixteen law schools, and received fifteen rejection letters. But on this day, I received a big envelope from the Florida A&M University College of Law—the main campus was in Tallahassee, but the law school had recently opened a branch in Orlando, Florida. I opened the mail, and started screaming right there in the post office. I finally got my first acceptance letter into law school. A day later, I reached out to the Council on Legal Education Opportunity (CLEO). I had previously connected with Mrs. Thomasine Williams, who was the director of admissions, but I could not get into CLEO without a law school. Now that I had a law school, I immediately called Mrs. Williams and gave her the news. A day later, Mrs. Williams informed me that she was admitting me into the 2006 CLEO Summer Institute at Thomas Jefferson School of Law, in San Diego, CA. Needless to say, in April 2006, I gave Deloitte my two weeks' notice, and left my job as a technology professional to pursue my dream of attending law school. First stop, Thomas Jefferson School of Law (TJSL) in San Diego!

I arrived in San Diego, and TJSL, in June 2006. They housed all of us in co-op residence halls at San Diego State University. The program's layout was much like the Summer Bridge Program from my college days at the University of Illinois. It was a six-week summer program, which introduced incoming minority law students to the rigors of law school. We took a condensed and intense introductory class in Contracts, Constitutional Law ("Con Law"), and Legal Writing. Naturally, legal writing, under Joe Bodine, my writing instructor, was my favorite course. Joe thought my writing was powerful. My ability to draft a *first, rough draft* of a legal memorandum was very impressive, even though I had never done it before. I just needed to polish my memo and learn how to incorporate the closed memo assignment cases.

The program was challenging, but it seemed that some counselors within the program purposefully exacerbated how hard it was by stressing out my colleagues/fellow students—more than was necessary. Naturally, I spoke up and

• brought it to the attention of the program directors at TJSL. I merely told them that I would rather be sent home than to continue watching the counselors behave in this way during our exam sessions, causing one or more of my classmates to miss out on the school of their choice, or any law school. I had a law school, so I had nothing to lose by taking such a hardline stance. The message got through to all staff members. They were sympathetic to the student's stress levels. We all survived CLEO and made it into our respective law schools in the Fall of 2006.

I started my journey at Florida A&M University College of Law in Orlando in August 2006. When I arrived in Orlando, I was less than impressed. But this was 100% my fault. The school had its challenges as a provisionally accredited law school at the time. But I used that as an excuse not to do what I was supposed to do. I survived my first year at FAMU, but the entire time, I had my heart set on going to the University of Miami (UM) School of Law in Coral Gables, Florida. Unfortunately, I did not have the grades to be admitted as a regular student. But I was admitted to UM as a visiting student and hoped that I could earn my way into the law school that way. During my year at UM Law School, I did well, but my efforts were not good enough to be admitted as a regular student. Additionally, a new administration had taken over at FAMU. So, although I could go back to FAMU, they would not allow me to transfer any of the UM core courses that were required courses at FAMU.

Not only was I devastated, but I was also embarrassed, frustrated, and pissed off. I was embarrassed because I now had to go back to the law school that I basically trashed to anyone that would listen. I was pissed because the school had a policy, unbeknownst to me, that you could NOT take any courses on FAMU's required course list at another institution. They had to be taken at FAMU, which meant that only the elective courses taken at UM would transfer over *IF* I were to return to FAMU. I did not know what to do. I was not ready to go back to Orlando, admit defeat, and humble myself before the FAMU administration. So, I just sat out the Fall semester of what would have been my third year of law school. Instead, I decided to stay in Miami for the Fall 2008 semester and continue working at the UM Athletic Department. I was only making minimum wage, and ultimately, did not have money to pay rent. I was getting some help from my mother, who was also pissed at me for opting not to go back to law school that semester. She did not care where I finished law school, or what it took. She just wanted me to finish, take and pass the bar exam in Illinois.

Money was extremely tight. I barely survived through the Fall and Winter months. But by the time December came around, I realized that I would have to go back to law school and finish what I started. I could not continue living the way I did—stressed out, broke, and unable to find work that would pay a decent salary in Miami. Miami was not a city that you could have an average job and make more than fifty thousand dollars a year. You either had to be an athlete, a celebrity, or an attorney to have a chance at a decent living. The cost of living was too high. And because everyone wanted to live in South Florida, the employment market did not bode well for regular people, with regular jobs. I had no choice but to humble myself, and accept that if I wanted to go back to law school, which at the time meant going back to FAMU, I would have to retake those courses I took at UM that were on the FAMU required course list. I finally got my mind ready to face the music and return to FAMU during the Winter 2009 semester. I registered online for courses and made plans to move my things out of the condo in Miami. But out of nowhere, just before making that final commitment to head back to Orlando, I discovered another option—John Marshall Law School in Atlanta, Georgia.

John Marshall was another ABA provisionally accredited school.[6] I applied to John Marshall, got accepted, and immediately had options. I met with the Registrar, Cheryl Ferebee, to determine what courses will transfer over if I choose to study at John Marshall instead of FAMU. They allowed my Evidence and Property courses to transfer over, but I had to retake Torts, Criminal Procedure, and Constitutional Law, and take the other required courses (Sales and Secured Transactions, Remedies, etc.). I prayed about it for several days and decided to go back to Atlanta and attend John Marshall.

---

6   It is now fully accredited.

My first semester at John Marshall was almost my last se-mester. I had only registered for four courses—one of which was Sales and Secured Transactions. I failed that course, which caused my GPA for the semester to fall below a 2.0. Thus, due to my poor academic performance, I was dis-missed from the law school. I appealed to the Dean of Stu-dents, but my appeal was denied. I had one appeal left before the Dean of the law school. I poured my heart out in a letter to the Dean, vowing to be a better student. The Dean ulti-mately granted my petition for reinstatement, citing that one semester of law school was not enough to evaluate my aca-demic ability. I was admitted under academic probation and had to meet with the Director of Academic Success, Kimber-ly D'Haene every week. I was happy not only to be reinstat-ed, but that Professor D'Haene was a black woman from the UM, where my mother was an alumnus as well.

My law school grades from that point on were much bet-ter. I was able to get off academic probation. In December 2010, I finally got my law degree. We did not have a gradu-ation ceremony during the Winter, so I did not walk or *Step Across the Stage* until May 2011. When I got my diploma, I held it for 20 minutes in the registrar's office and broke down in tears. I went across the street to the FedEx Office. It was windy that day, and the diploma flew out of my hand and out into the middle of Peachtree Road. Luckily, one of my classmates was there to secure it without incident. I scanned it onto a flash drive and posted it on Facebook. I was so happy. But there was still so much work to do. Getting my law degree was one thing, but I still had to pass the bar.

After graduating, I began preparing for the Illinois Bar Exam. Initially, I had planned to move to D.C. after law school and sit for the Maryland exam. But my mother, in all her infinite wisdom, kept urging me to sit for the Illinois Bar Exam instead. At the time, I had no plans to come back to Chicago. Little did I know that GOD had his own plan for me.

I went ahead and registered for the February 2011 administration of the Illinois Bar Exam. I took the BARBRI prep course for Illinois remotely from my apartment in Atlanta, Georgia. I also stayed and watched the BARBRI lessons at the John Marshall Law School Library. I went to Chicago to sit for the exam at the Gleason Center in downtown Chicago in February 2011. I missed passing the exam by three points. I reregistered for the Illinois Bar Exam in July that same year, and missed passing that exam by five points.

I also started working as a contract document review attorney in Richmond, Virginia, and Washington D.C. for six months. Every day, I would commute back and forth from Washington D.C., where I stayed with my D.C. mother, Sandra Craft, to Richmond—an hour and a half down I-95. Later, I retook the bar exam again February 2012 and failed miserably by double digit points. At that point, I decided that I would take a break for a while.

In December 2011, I was hired at North Carolina A&T State University, in Greensboro, North Carolina, as the Assistant Athletic Director for Compliance. A month before I left for Greensboro, Karen, Amber's mother, and I had reconnected. I hated leaving her and Amber all over again. I was trying to spend as much time in Atlanta as possible. Karen was incredibly supportive of me being in Greensboro, and never made that an issue. But even when I was in Greensboro, my mind was clearly in Atlanta. It would not be long before my time at North Carolina A&T would come to an end. I could not adjust to what they called the "Aggie Way". To me, the Aggie Way, was simply an excuse not to achieve excellence. Excellence that I had become accustomed to working in previous athletic positions with the University of Illinois, University of Miami, and Georgia Tech. I only remained in "Aggieland" for three months before resigning. For several reasons, I needed to move back to Atlanta. However, I had no plan of action of what I was going to do, or how I was going to support myself, Karen, and Amber, once I got there.

CHAPTER 3

'GOD is not as concerned about our comfort as
He is our purpose. Sometimes He shakes things up to
get us to our destiny.'

—Joel Osteen

Martin Luther King Jr once said that, 'the ultimate measure
of a man is not where he stands in moments of comfort and
convenience, but where he stands at times of challenge and
controversy.' Well, 2012 was seemingly filled with several
moments of challenge and controversy—it was the year I was
forced to become a man and step out on my own. After leaving what many considered a dream job as the Assistant Athletic Director for Compliance at North Carolina A&T State
University in Greensboro, North Carolina, I was faced with
the reality of unemployment, and homelessness. I was cut off
financially from my parents. At the same time, I was trying
to save face and prove to the woman that I loved that I could
step up and provide the security that she needed, and a
home to lay her head at night, even if I didn't have a place of
my own. 2012 for me was definitely a year for growth,
maturity, and priorities.

After leaving Greensboro, I headed back to Atlanta. While searching for jobs in the Atlanta area, I did not list on my resume, that I had graduated from law school because I did not want to be categorized as "overqualified". I needed a job and money. But most importantly, I needed to get off the road, and be physically based in Atlanta. I started doing document review jobs again in Charlotte, North Carolina and Columbia, South Carolina. I worked for about three months before I found an IT job back in Atlanta. Throughout my employment search, I did not have a place to live. Before leaving for Greensboro, I told Karen that she and Amber could just move into my apartment in Atlanta. That was before I decided that I was only going to be in Greensboro for two months.

When I made the decision to quit my job and return, they had already moved in. Although Karen and I had started dating again, we agreed not to cohabitate while Amber was still in the house. Because of the document review projects I was working on across state lines in North and South Carolina, I was not home during the week, and would only come home every other weekend. They say absence makes the heart grow fonder. The only thing that helped Karen and I, was that I stayed away for days on end, and occasionally, weeks at a time. I would often stay in extended stay hotels or use my hotel points for a night or two and stay at the Hyatt Place. But most times, in an effort to save money, I would just work all day, and sleep in my truck. At the time, I had a 2003 Ford Explorer that I slept in many nights, in various hotel parking lots in Columbia (SC).

There was a girl from Philadelphia, Mandisa, who traveled all the way to Columbia because she could not get a job back home. She was in the same predicament as I was—could not get a job because she was still trying to pass the bar. We exchanged stories, only to find out that she was sleeping in her car as well. She also had a Gold's Gym membership ,and would head there to shower in the morning before heading into the review center. We hung out a few times to get our minds off our situation. Occasionally, I would commute to Charlotte and spend the night at Sabrina's house, my cousin who lived in Charlotte. I was happy to have a couch to crash on versus my truck. And I loved spending time with my then baby cousins, Landon and Logan. But I was afraid that I would eventually wear out my welcome like I had done before. Eventually, I made the decision that I could not do it anymore—I had to go back to Atlanta.

I signed up with a staffing agency for tech jobs. The staffing agency got me an interview for a temp-to-perm IT position with General Electric (GE) in their Retail Finance Group. During the interview process, I did not tell them that I had a law degree. I needed a job in Atlanta. I was offered the position with GE, but the salary was extremely low. Moreover, despite having a job in Atlanta, there was still the issue that Amber was still at home, and Karen did not want us living together.

The GE office was on Windward Parkway in Alpharetta, Georgia, right next to the Hilton Garden Inn. I would go to work for as long as I could, get something to eat after work, and slept in the hotel parking lot. Usually, I would just crash in the front seat of my 2003 Ford Explorer, and recline the seat all the way back. Occasionally, I would curl up in the back seat, so that I could stretch my legs a bit. During this time, I was sad, lonely, and depressed. I did not want Karen knowing that I was sleeping in my truck. I could not tell her that I did not have a place to go. But I'm sure deep down that she knew. She just did not want to crush my fragile ego any more than it already had been. I would sleep until about 5am, which was when the LA Fitness down the street opened. I maintained my LA Fitness membership, so I could use the facilities to shower and workout before going to work every day.

Around Amber's high school graduation, my friend Khadiyah ("Kay") Lewis called to check on me one day. At the time, she was leasing this massive house in Dunwoody—it was basically a HUGE mansion. When she realized that I did not have a place to stay, she offered me one of the guest bedrooms. Immediately, that lifted a huge weight lifted off my shoulders. The truck had served its purpose, but I was so ready to have a bed, with a TV. I could finally watch the NBA playoffs in a house, instead of sitting at one of the local bars until I got sleepy and tired. That lasted about a month because she was moving into a one-bedroom apartment. Shortly afterwards, Kay landed a role on VH1's *Love and Hip-Hop Atlanta*. Before leaving the house, I remembered that my friend, Monique, and her dad owned a condo in the Hill Street Lofts, which was not too far from Turner Field. The

Atlanta neighborhood near Turner Field, where the Braves played their home games before relocating to Cobb County, is straight hood. But the Hill Street Lofts was a gated community, I had a parking space, and it was a temporary place for me to lay my head until it was time for Amber to go to college at Georgia State University and move into the dorms.

In September 2012, Karen, and I finally moved in together, as roommates and in separate bedrooms in the apartment. At first, it was weird that we slept in separate bedrooms. We would have sex like savages, only to then sleep in our separate rooms—like boxers going to their separate corners. Amber would come home every now and then, and just sleep in Karen's room. Just when I thought things would be okay between us, the month of October 2012 rolled around. As if anything else bad could have happened that year, we got evicted from the apartment. That was totally my fault. I was stalling on paying the rent, trying to stack cash, which is NOT a good thing to do. We did not get evicted because I did not have the rent money—we got evicted because I was stupid and careless. There was an issue between my bank and the online rent payment system. I had never been late before, but I was late with the September payment, which I had planned to pay in October. But the Marshalls came to execute the eviction order before I could pay the October rent.

When I attempted to pay the rent that day, the office manager, Rachel, who was my friend, called me frantically saying that the Marshalls were there to evict us if I did not pay rent. I had money in a Fidelity account that I could only access online, and was linked to a debit card. At the time, other than the Fidelity account, I only had an account at the Coca-Cola Federal Credit Union, with no debit card (ATM card only) linked to that account. So, I would have to wire funds from my credit union account, to my Fidelity account, to have money on a card that I could use like a credit card. We did not have that much time to settle all this out.

The apartment complex had a new property manager. I had the money on a Fidelity debit card. However, the property manager would not let me pay with a debit/credit card for fear that the payment could be reversed. We had dogs in the apartment. Miles and Nina (twin Pekingese dogs), and Scooter (who was rambunctious and chased his own tail around all day). Nina had just given birth to four puppies. The Marshalls let me secure the dogs, and then the leasing company's "eviction crew" began putting our stuff into trash bags and placing them out on the curb. I was so embarrassed. The hard part was that I had to call Karen at work, and tell her that we were getting evicted. I sucked it up, swallowed my pride and made the call. I told her that she needed to come home because we were getting evicted. Karen was obviously furious... actually, she was pissed! She immediately left work to come to the house and sit and watch all our stuff being put out on the street while I went to secure a storage unit. I asked my friend Demetrius to come sit with her, and watch our stuff, while I went to get a moving truck. Karen did not tell anyone about what happened, but she did not speak to me for days after that. She ended up going to stay with her brother Keith, and I ended up staying a couple of days with my baby sister, Erica, for the weekend, before moving over to the Holiday Inn on Camp Creek later that week.

As luck would have it, one of my good friends, Kendric, who ironically had just evicted a tenant from his home, gave me a chance. Even though he knew my situation, he allowed me to rent his house— on the strength of us being friends. We got evicted that Friday, but I signed the lease and moved all of our stuff into the new place that following Friday. To her credit, Karen never told her parents, and most importantly, she never told our daughter Amber about us getting evicted because of my stupidity and lack of follow-up. All Amber and Karen's parents knew was that we moved out of the apartment, and into a house.

As it turns out, we got the house just in time. Karen was scheduled to have fibroids surgery in January. After her surgery, the doctor showed us the fibroids. One was the size of a softball, and the other two were like miniature golf balls. The doctor told us that if we were considering having another child, that soon after Karen recovered would be the time to do it. The doctor also looked at me and said that Karen's sex drive would likely be off the charts, "so be ready!" That was hilarious to me. Karen stayed in the hospital for two days after the surgery. I stayed right there by her side, curling up in a chair when it was time for me to go to sleep—only going home to feed and let the dogs out occasionally.

Karen initially went to her parents while she was recovering. But when she came back to the house, the doctor was right, her sex drive had increased significantly. Not that it was lacking before, but this time more often, she was initiating things. Karen stayed at the house for about another month, while she was waiting on the rehab work at her parent's old house in College Park. They had been renting it out to another tenant, but ended up giving the tenant notice and allowing Karen and Amber to move in, where they still reside today.

In 2014, another moment of truth was starting to present itself. My brother, Kris, had moved to Georgia, and I moved in with him for a while, letting the house I was renting go. Kris had rented this huge house in Locust Grove, Georgia, about 40 minutes south of Atlanta. The goal was to hopefully save some money by moving in with him. I was behind on my car payments on a 2013 Ford Fusion I had purchased just a year earlier. I thought I could avoid paying the lender simply because they had no idea where to find me.

A few months after moving in, Kris told me he was moving back to Chicago. He had only moved to Atlanta to be closer to his daughter. But as it turned out, his daughter Kristen, and her mother, Kierra, were planning to relocate back to Chicago. Kris had a friend, who had also decided to relocate back to Chicago and was looking for someone to take over her lease in East Atlanta. I jumped at the opportunity to move back into the city. So, I moved my things into the apartment, and kept my Ford Fusion in the parking garage.

I figured I was safe from a repossession because the parking garage was private. I had no idea that the garage had a contract with a local tow company to scour the parking lot at night to remove illegally parked vehicles.

As luck would have it, technology had changed by then, and I did not realize that tow truck drivers could now scan VIN numbers to identify vehicles that were out for repossession. Turns out my car was on that list and it was repossessed in the middle of the night. I did not even find out until the next morning when I was getting ready to go to the barbershop to get my haircut—SMH! Eventually, I found a guy on Craigslist who was moving out of state and was leasing a brand-new Honda Accord. I paid him five hundred dollars and was supposed to send him five hundred dollars per month, every month after that, until the car was paid in full. But the guy disappeared, and I just kept the car, without making any more payments. Eventually, I bought a 2013 Nissan Maxima at a 'buy here, pay here' dealership. The car had a cutoff switch, that had to be renewed every two weeks after I made my payment. That process helped my credit because I was forced to make payments on time.

While all of this was going on, I caught myself trying to impress Karen, so that we could get back together. We had our annual trip to Mexico scheduled for the first week in September—a trip that I hoped would rekindle our romantic relationship. It turned out to be not so great because Karen was not feeling me. She knew I was drowning financially, and that I was a complete mess. Even though we stayed in Mexico for six days, we might as well have been sleeping in separate rooms.

When we got back from Mexico, our mutual friend, George, told me that he asked Karen if we had a romantic time, as we had done in the past. He told me that Karen's response was simply that I needed to get my sh*t together—we, again, did not speak for a month or two after that. When I left the airport, even though I was crushed and probably at my lowest point ever, I drove four hours to Gainesville, Florida, to temporarily live with my law school classmate, McArthur Shelton. Unlike myself, McArthur, or "Mac", had passed the Florida Bar. However, he was a full-time teacher in Gainesville, his hometown. He also represented the local teacher's union as their labor attorney. I was still working with the Active Directory team with GE remotely, so I had money coming in. I offered to pay him rent, but he told me not to worry about it, and just do what I needed to do to get myself together. That was a load lifted off my shoulders, allowed me to save up money for the first time in a while, and not live paycheck to paycheck.

I stayed in Gainesville for about two months. I was on a sabbatical from the rest of the world. I did not get a haircut until I traveled to Atlanta for the Chicago Bears vs. Atlanta Falcons game in October that year. Of course, I told Karen that I would be in town that weekend, but she was not interested. The game was a release for me because Otha, my best friend, came to town. I had a chance to spend time, and destress, with my friends who had no idea what I was going through. After the game, I went back to Gainesville and stayed for another month. But while I was there, I had an epiphany. I was finally sick and tired of being sick and tired. I realized that there was only one way I could dig myself out of this rut that I had been in for the better part of the year. I had to take another shot at the Illinois Bar Exam.

It was time for me to emerge permanently from my two-month sabbatical in Gainesville. I was ready and it was time. In November 2014, I said goodbye to Mac and thanked him for having my back when I needed it the most. I hit the road on I-75 and headed back to Atlanta. One of my classmates from law school had introduced me to one of her childhood friends who had a house in South Fulton County, in Atlanta. As luck would have it, Karen, who also sold real estate in Atlanta, actually sold him that house. Oddly enough, my ex-girlfriend, Kiya, now married, lived just two doors down with her husband. I rented the first-floor master bedroom from him for four hundred dollars per month. The room was just as large as a studio apartment. When I returned, Karen agreed to meet me for dinner at this Mexican restaurant that was close to where we both lived. Amber and I had been communicating over the previous two months about how I could make a splash with her mother. Karen had a thing for shoes. So, we decided on some red Jimmy Choo shoes that I surprised Karen with at dinner. I ordered them from my friend, Mack Jones, who worked at the Neiman Marcus in Lenox Mall in Atlanta's Buckhead neighborhood.

At dinner, Karen shared that she had decided to go back to school. I told her that I was proud of her and that I would do anything I could to help her. I was not planning on giving her the shoes until Christmas, but I felt this was as good a time as any to give them to her. So, I went to my car, and returned with the gift box containing the shoes and gave them to her. Karen nearly had an orgasm when she saw the shoes. She told me that she thought I was buying her some Jimmy Choo perfume when she initially saw the box. At the same time, I told her that I was going back to finish what I started and pass the Illinois Bar Exam in February 2015. I did not think it would bring us back together, but I finally did have her attention.

In January 2015, I started prepping for the bar exam. I took the Kaplan prep course for the Illinois Exam. I did not focus at all on Karen—I blocked her out and focused on my studies. Although she checked in on me every now and then, I was laser-focused. I convinced my mother to pay for the Kaplan bar review course on my behalf. I was still working my Active Directory Job with GE overnight, so I was able to watch the lessons, and study, every day from my room. I completed and uploaded the daily assignments I needed to submit so that I could pass the bar—something the Kaplan course promised if I did everything the lessons required. In February 2015, I traveled to Chicago three days before the exam. I stayed at the Crowne Plaza on North Halsted Avenue, down the street from the UIC Forum, where I was to take the exam. On day one of the exam, I felt great. I felt like I rocked the essay portion of the exam.

However, day two was a different story. Unexpectedly, I came down with the flu. It impacted my performance during the morning session. I was so sick that the person sitting next to me asked to move to another seat. I could not blame them—this was an important exam. During the break, I went across the street to the Jewel Osco pharmacy to get some over the counter meds to help me get through the exam. I had to take the meds prior to coming back to the examination room. The Illinois bar examiners had a rule that required examinees to get prior permission or advance approval to bring meds into the examination room. Apparently, I was supposed to know on December 31st, 2014, when I registered for the exam, that I would be sick during the exam—but I digress.

After the exam, I went back to my hotel room and just went to bed. I ended up staying an extra night because I was too sick to travel. The next day, Vivian came to visit me—that was the first time I had seen her in years. We went for dinner at Giordano's on Halsted and Van Buren. At that time, I had a strained relationship with my mother and stepfather as well. So, I had not seen or spoken to any of them since my mom's sixtieth birthday party in Jamaica—that Karen and I attended. Vivian gave me a ride back to my hotel. Before she left, I told her that I loved her and gave her some advice. I told her to be better than me, and not to do anything to fall out of favor with my parents—just like I had done. A month later, I received my results back from the 2015 Illinois Bar Exam. I opened the letter and unfortunately, I'd failed again. The next day, I received my score report via email—this time, I had missed passing the exam by five freaking points.

CHAPTER 4

'Your imagination is your preview of life's
coming attractions.'

—Albert Einstein

At this point, I began to realize that, for my own good, that
GOD had been orchestrating things in my life—even some
of my relationships, and friendships. That is why it is not sur-
prising that he sent Courtney Bell into my life. We met in
2016. I was introduced to Courtney by a mutual friend of
ours. At the time, I was still living in Atlanta, but planning on
moving back to Chicago. Courtney was a talented writer, Life
Coach, and managed several college programs at Columbia
College. She also taught courses at various community colleges in Chicago.

To me, Courtney was truly the *bomb*. I knew that if
I wanted to be with her, I had to step up my game. Courtney and I had great attraction and passion for each other.
The sex was f*cking amazing. Mmmph… mmmph, just the
thought of it still entices my imagination. The best part was
that she was into me, and I felt it. Even though I was still
going through a financial transition period, she believed in

me. She was a great motivator and made me want to be a better man. Courtney was unlike any woman I had ever dated before. Most importantly, she knew I was going through a rough time, and was not judgmental at all.

As much as Karen had a hold on my heart still, I was all in when it came to Courtney Bell, and truly, truly thought she was going to be the one. Courtney was *badass*, and all her friends were doctors, psychologists, lawyers, etc. Courtney was very instrumental in getting me to the finish line and encouraged me to retake the Illinois Bar Exam. She encouraged me to take advantage of the opportunity that I was presented with. My mother, stepfather, and I had made peace and moved on from the past. I borrowed money from my stepfather to pay for my BARBRI prep courses. At this time, they had agreed to house me in one of their vacant apartments in the 18-unit building that they owned across the street from the University of Chicago campus. I did not have to pay rent, and I did not have to work—I just needed to study and pass this bar exam once and for all.

As always, the bar preparatory course (BARBRI) began in January at Chicago-Kent Law School. It was the Spring Exam, so the lectures were not live, but they were on video. Getting up and traveling to Kent Law School daily gave me the structure I needed to properly prepare for the exam. On the day before Martin Luther King Jr. holiday, Courtney and I got into an argument that ultimately led to our breakup. I was devastated because I was really feeling her. I believed that we were a power couple unlike any other, and that we could have come together to truly make some entrepreneurial money. I tried several times to get back with her, but she was not having it. I was still chasing my dream and she was looking for a partner that was already established.

I had lost my focus, and my studies were noticeably suffering. The bar exam had taken a back seat to all my distraught emotions of losing Courtney—at least temporarily. My studying and preparation came to a screeching halt. I was clearly upset because I absolutely loved Courtney, and like I said, I thought we had the potential to be the perfect power couple. I could not get her out of my mind. She made me want to step my game up to match her level of expectation. The argument was so bad that Courtney stopped accepting my calls, and even blocked my number. However, about three weeks before the exam, I received a card in the mail from Courtney. Prior to us breaking up, she had me make her a promise. She made me promise that I would pass my bar exam no matter what happened between us. The card Courtney sent said, "Remember your promise to me. Congratulations in advance on passing the bar exam." The card reignited a fire in me. After that, I regained my initial steam and focus. I resumed my studies and used the remaining time to prepare.

I was a regular at the Kent Law School library, and even asked a friend of mine, who had passed the bar exam years ago, to meet me after class at the law school to share some of her tips on how to pass the exam. She stressed the importance of not learning the law but figuring out how to take the test and pass the exam. As the days grew closer to the February 2017 exam, the weather was unseasonably warm—temperatures were in the high 60s and low 70s. About two days before the exam, I texted Katreshia, my former boss at North Carolina AT&T State University. She was the only reason why it was difficult for me to leave Greensboro. She had worked so hard and been so instrumental in paving the way to get me to Greensboro, and I felt like I let her down. I was so happy that she reached out a few years ago. It meant so much to me that we could move on. Anyway, she had also been planning to sit for the bar exam in Georgia. I texted her that I was taking the exam one more time. Katreshia texted back #thelasttime. Tears instantly brimmed in my eyes. More than anyone, she knew how much I needed to pass this exam to have any sort of life worth living. I was almost inconsolable, but I got myself together and finished my studying for the day.

Remember when I took the exam in February 2015, it was so cold that I got sick on the second day of the exam with the flu. They would not let me take any medication into the testing room because I did not make prior arrangements to accommodate my request, as required. I remember thinking how the f*ck was I supposed to know that I would catch the flu on day two of the exam? I ended up failing that exam by 5 points. When you pass, they do not tell you your score. They send you a score report which breaks down how you did on day one (essay portion) versus day two (multiple choice). I did excellent on day one. On day 2, the day I was sick, I did not do so well on the multiple-choice section—otherwise known as the "MBE". This time, I knew it would be different. It had to be, otherwise I could not see myself taking it again.

By the time February 21st and 22nd, 2017 came around, I was ready. I was determined that this time would be the last time I sat for the exam. Instead of staying in the hotel, as my mother recommended, I decided to commute to the exam from home. On day one, in the morning, I took an Uber to take the exam and requested that the driver drop me off at the bus station across the street from the UIC Forum. I was about 45 minutes early, so I just sat there looking at the building's exterior. I posted a picture of the building on social media, thanking everyone for putting up with me throughout this journey, and letting everyone know that this time, the final time, I was more prepared than ever. The weather was extremely warm on both days—unseasonably warm for February (high 60s). I took the exam on both days—this time with no health issues. I felt good about the exam, but I had this uncertainty nagging at me before I got my results— which had always been there. Since this was the February exam, February applicants received their results no later than April 1st, 2017.

On the morning of March 31st, 2017, at 8:30am, I received an email that the Illinois Bar Examiners had posted the exam results to our profile pages. I was so nervous—I knew I could not afford to fail, but I also knew I did not have the energy to retake the exam if, in fact, I failed again. Before sitting down, I walked from my bedroom to the computer office/den, while saying a prayer. When I was situated in my office chair, I logged into my examinee page and said one more prayer before opening the results. I had opened this same email/letter six times in the past, and the first line usually read: 'We regret to advise you that you have failed the 20XX Administration of the Illinois Bar Exam.' I was cautiously optimistic as I clicked on the letter. Then, I said one more prayer and opened it. As I opened the message, there it was—I could not believe it. I was not sure that I was reading it correctly when I did not see the words "We regret to advise you ..." Instead of "regret", I saw the word "pleased". So, I continued reading the first line of the letter: 'Dear Mr. Eason: We are **_pleased_** to advise that you have passed...' That is all I read before losing it. I mean I absolutely lost it! I started shouting as loud as I could, "YES!! THANK YOU, LORD!" multiple times—mind you it was 8:30am, but I did not care. My next-door neighbor, Nyahne, told me later she could hear me shouting through the walls. She did not know why at the time, but the only thing that kept her from walking over to make sure I was alright was that she could tell that my screams were obviously screams and tears of joy. I was overly ecstatic and excited. I had finally passed the Illinois Bar Exam.

I immediately called my mother in tears. When she answered the phone, I was still crying. She could not understand what was wrong because I was not saying anything, I was just crying. She was driving back home to Michigan

City from Chicago apparently. I finally calmed down and just read the first sentence of the letter. When my mother heard the words indicating that I had finally passed the Illinois Bar Exam, all she could do was scream out loudly over the phone, "*HALLELUJAH*"!! It was as if her prayers had been answered as well.

I finally called Karen and Amber via Facetime. Amber was still asleep, but Karen was getting ready for work. Like my mother, Karen, too, was confused, because she did not know what was wrong or why I was asking for Amber's whereabouts. All she saw was that my face looked like I had been crying. She asked what was wrong. I told her "nothing" and just read the letter to her. When I got to the part about me passing the 2017 Illinois bar exam, she screamed out, "YAAAAAAY!!" Then, I got on Facebook and went live, still crying, and shared my joy for passing the bar with my followers. I read the first part of the letter via Facebook Live. On that day, my post received over 500 likes—the most I had ever received. I had finally done it. I passed the Illinois bar exam! It had taken seven years and seven tries. Although I had previously failed the exam six times, none of that mattered anymore. The seventh time was the charm. I finally passed. I tried calling Courtney the day that I got my results, but the phone went to voice mail. I saw her a few weeks later at the cleaners that we both frequent on 22nd and Michigan in the South Loop neighborhood of Chicago. There was so much I wanted to say to her – namely, thank you. I always felt that we cut short what could have been an amazing relationship.

On June 27th, 2017, the dream was complete. I was sworn in before the Illinois Supreme Court and admitted to practice law in the state of Illinois. I officially became "Marques A. Eason, Esq.," and the legend of "Big Daddy Esquire" was born. I contemplated inviting Courtney to my swearing-in ceremony downtown. But I wasn't certain that she would come. However, I was well represented, as a lot of my family and friends were at the Federal Courthouse in downtown Chicago that morning. Of course, I learned later that had I asked, she would've definitely come.

In October 2018, Courtney and I met for drinks at a bowling alley on the University of Chicago campus in Hyde Park. That was the first time I got to say everything that I had been dying to tell her; specifically, the role that she played in my life at that time, what an inspiration she was to me and how much I missed her and missed having the opportunity to truly see what we could have been. That night, we shared this amazing, passionate kiss. Our goodbye kisses were always passionate and truly the sh*t. Soon afterward, we briefly started dating again. But for all the passion we shared, it just was not meant to be. At least this time, I felt like we both tried our best, but we just fell short. I still love her today for everything that she was to me during that season of my life. Courtney was the ultimate motivator for me, and GOD put her in my life to serve a purpose. GOD specifically positioned her to get me over that hump of passing the Illinois bar exam.

Courtney and I have not kept in touch since then. But every year, on the anniversary of me getting sworn in (June 27th), I make it a point to send Courtney an email or a text message, thanking her for pushing me. Were it not for her, I may have never done what I thought was unattainable, after failing several times. I finally passed, and I have no problem stating as fact that, outside of GOD, I owe Courtney Bell for finally pushing me to accomplish what had taken over a decade to complete.

PRESENT

'The more anger towards the past you carry in your heart, the less capable you are of loving in the present.'

—**Barbara De Angelis**

CHAPTER 5

'In dark places, we prove to GOD what
we are really made of. You have to be faithful when
things are not going your way'

—Joel Osteen

After I was sworn in, I decided to establish my own law practice on the South Side of Chicago, in my old neighborhood of Beverly, specializing in family law, real estate, and probate. Things were on the rise for me. In 2018, I made a hundred and seventy-three thousand dollars ($173,000.00) in the first year of my solo practice, and nearly two hundred and fifty thousand ($250,000.00) dollars in the second year. It was a good start and a pivotal moment for me, and my career. I was just putting my stamp as an attorney in the Chicago real estate market. In addition to that, my oldest daughter, Amber, had launched her solo music career, and I was her manager. We were starting the year 2020 right with my birthday bash! Amber flew out to Chicago to perform at my party, and I was ready to finish off 2020 with nothing but good vibes and positive energy. Her mother, Karen came as well because this was Amber's first performance in Chicago, but we kept that a secret from Amber. I also secretly arranged to have her boyfriend, Jared, come as well. That night was amazing and capped off an incredible weekend. If you had told me that my life was about to dramatically change because of a deadly virus that would sweep through this entire world, I would have probably not believed you.

The coronavirus or COVID-19 is a disease that attacks the respiratory system. It is believed that the virus originated out of a lab in Wuhan, China in late 2019, and gradually made its way to foreign countries, and ultimately, the United States. Common symptoms of the coronavirus include fever, cough, fatigue, shortness of breath, and loss of smell. Complications may include pneumonia and acute respiratory distress syndrome. The time from exposure to onset of symptoms is typically around five days.

The Center for Disease Control (CDC) in Atlanta had issued guidelines regarding common symptoms and the measures people should take to prevent infection: washing your hands, covering one's mouth while coughing, maintaining a distance of at least six feet ("Social Distancing"), wearing a mask while out in public settings, and self-isolation for people who are symptomatic. The problem was that it was still very new to us in the U.S. When the first wave came to the states, no one was prepared. Not to mention, it did not help that President Trump held multiple press conferences downplaying the seriousness of the virus. His lackadaisical response did not impact me in any way because I do not listen to Trump, or his radical and ridiculous statements that he seems to make far too frequently.

Government authorities responded by implementing travel restrictions, instituting stay at home orders, and lockdowns. The pandemic also led to the postponement or cancellation of sporting, religious, political, and cultural events nationwide. As I write this book, schools, universities, and colleges are closed, and/or have adopted remote learning models in over 185 countries, including the United States of America.

The coronavirus hit the African American and Latino populations the hardest. In my opinion, at the beginning, African Americans did not seriously heed the government's warnings. Rumors and stigmas swirled among the younger population that this virus only affected white people and the older population. This was far from the case. African Americans, or Blacks, had the highest rate of coronavirus related deaths in Chicago.[7] People of color seemed to be impacted the most by the coronavirus, and the number of deaths attributed to the coronavirus.

When news first broke about the coronavirus being discovered, I just remember hoping that it did not come to the United States. But other than that, I never gave too much thought about it—let alone whether there was a possibility I could catch it. On or about March 13th, 2020, an NBA game between Utah Jazz and Memphis Grizzles was canceled due

---

7 https://www.chicagotribune.com/coronavirus/ct-coronavirus-chicago-health-disparities-data-20200410-rf7lmmvgurf-wxpxiatebsozwsu-story.html

to Jazz forward Rudy Gobert testing positive for the virus. Then, my thoughts changed slightly. I started thinking that this virus was getting too close. I hoped I would not catch this virus. Never did I, in my wildest dreams, think that I would live in a world where a pandemic would change our way of life as we knew it, or that by March 13th, 2020, the coronavirus was already incubating in my system.

In my lifetime, I have never seen such an epidemic or pandemic that would literally bring the world to a halt. My favorite sports—football, baseball, and basketball—were either delayed, canceled, or postponed. The impact this pandemic has had on the economy was unforeseeable. Restaurants were forced to provide take-out only services; small businesses (namely barbershops, hair and nail salons, and many others) were forced to close for a period of time. Many people lost their jobs, causing unemployment rates to climb to record numbers in most states. The physical, emotional, and financial impact of the coronavirus pandemic was real.

Unfortunately, like many, I believed that I was indestructible, or at least immune to having my life significantly impacted by something as serious as the coronavirus pandemic. From a spiritual point of view, Joel Osteen describes this pandemic as a "SHIFT" and described it as GOD shaking and shifting things to place us in a better position moving forward. And unimaginably, I became a living witness to this shift.

THE SHIFTING

Before I was infected, I never really had a major stint in a hospital. In February 2020, while visiting my daughter in Atlanta, Georgia, I felt dizzy and lightheaded as I got off the plane. I figured that once I got food in my system that it would go away. But that was not the case. I got to my hotel room and tried to sleep it off, but that did not work either. I could barely walk or stand—let alone use the bathroom—without getting dizzy. As I was waiting on Amber so that we could head out for her show rehearsal, I went downstairs and sat at the bar. I wanted desperately to get some food in my stomach. I ordered some catfish fingers—however, the smell of the fried catfish was just too much for me. I could not eat it, so I gave it back.

The bartender, who was a friend of mine, Warren, tried to give me some water. But just as Amber walked in, I threw that up as well. Amber asked if I was alright. I told her that I was, just so she would not worry. Even though it was just a rehearsal, I needed her to be on her "A" game that night. I went to the bathroom and got myself together. Afterwards, we took an Uber to the rehearsal studio. An hour into the rehearsal, I was still feeling dizzy. But I could at least sit up straight. At that time, Karen started blowing up our phones.

I texted Karen back and reminded her that we were in rehearsal. She responded that she had heard what happened to me at the bar. She found out from a friend of hers, who had a female friend that was working at that bar (that woman has friends all over the place). I told her, as I told Amber, I was alright because I did not want her to worry as well. But apparently, she had already sent a text to Amber, directing her to take me to the hospital when we were done with rehearsal. As soon as the rehearsal ended, Amber looked at me and said, "Mom says I gotta take you to the hospital." I sighed and was a bit irritated, but I said okay. I made a deal with Amber that we would take an Uber back to the hotel, and we would call 911 and wait for the paramedics to pick me up from there. I spent two nights in the hospital—I was diagnosed with a TIA, also known as a mini stroke. They treated me for high blood pressure, stabilized my levels, and I was released two days later, just in time to see my baby girl perform. I thought that was the end of my health challenges for the year 2020. Boy was I wrong by a longshot.

On Sunday, March 15th, 2020, I could feel what I thought was just a bad cold coming on. Nothing that made me think that I had contracted the coronavirus. I had just celebrated my birthday a week prior on Sunday, March 8th, 2020, at "Gametyme Sports Bar and Grill" in Lynwood, Illinois with Amber, Karen, and Jared. On the morning of March 16th, 2020, what I was feeling had become more than just a bad cold. I was extremely weak. I barely had enough strength to make it from my bed to the bathroom. I suffered from diarrhea. I was going to the bathroom every hour on the hour. When I could walk to my computer office/den, I could only sit up at my desk for a few minutes to send emails, but nothing significant, workwise. I had to keep lying back down after extended periods of time. I also noticed that I was extremely dehydrated.

I consulted with my primary care physician, and my parents' friend, Dr. Reuben Nichols. Based on the symptoms I was describing, he advised me to take Imodium D for the diarrhea, and drink either Pedialyte or Gatorade to get electrolytes into my system. But I knew it was more than that when I could not stand up long enough to do simple things like open the door or prepare food for myself. Things finally became serious enough that I needed to go to the hospital on March 18th, 2020.

My mother had asked Kris to come by my house and do a wellness check. I think Kris showed up around six or seven pm that night. When he arrived, he rang the bell several times and then started calling and texting my phone. I was in my bedroom asleep but woke up when he called my phone. I got up and tried to walk into the living room to get to the buzzer to open the downstairs door to let him in, but I was so weak that I ended up collapsing on the floor right in front of the door and before I could reach the buzzer. My phone was in my hand, so I sent him a text message to ring my next-door neighbor's doorbell because I could unlock my door from my phone.

Kris began to ring Nyahne's doorbell. At first, she was clueless about what was going on, and told Kris to stop ring-ing her doorbell. Kris then told her that he was my brother and that it was an emergency and asked her to buzz him in. Nyahne finally let him in, walked across the hall to my door. She opened the door and found me lying on the floor in front of the door. I was conscious the whole time. When Kris came upstairs, he helped me get up and lay down on the couch, while he called 911. After that, the fire department and paramedics came and wheeled me down the stairs to the ambulance and over to the University of Chicago main campus hospital in Hyde Park. As they were taking me downstairs, I realized that I did not have my charger or my other phone. The other phone was buried in my bed. But I never worried too much about it because I never thought I would be in the hospital for very long. The hospital was only a few blocks away from my building, and I remember it being cold outside and all I had on was a short sleeve Chicago Bears Khalil Mack t-shirt.

At this point, while I did not know what was wrong, or did not think what I was experiencing was life-threatening, I started thinking about my best friend O, and how he died so young at age 43. I began wondering if the same thing would happen to me. Would I survive? Would I see my house again? Would I see my daughters again? Would I ever get the chance to see my grandbaby, whom I still have yet to meet because of the difficult relationship between Vivian and I? So many questions, but still too early for answers at this point. At some point before Kris arrived, I posted on Facebook that I was not feeling well. I remember Amber had sent me a text message, asking me what was wrong. But I could not even respond. I was that weak that I could not answer my baby's text.

When we arrived at the hospital, the ER was a mad house of people waiting to be admitted. One of the U of C intake staff members was so annoyed with me because I could not describe my symptoms—all I knew was that I felt so sick. I just remember her getting up and saying that 'she could not do this tonight.' I certainly was not trying to be difficult. Considering I was sick, I was doing the best I could.

It was not until a couple of hours later, after being admitted, that doctors informed me that I had, in fact, tested positive for the coronavirus. Remember, how I kept saying that I hoped I would not catch the virus? Well, I did. The global pandemic that had already flatlined the U.S. economy and caused the deaths of many had now knocked on my front door. But I was not scared yet. I convinced myself that it was not as bad as it sounded. I figured they would keep me for a night or two, and send me home. Little did I know, the current state of my health had the doctors alarmed. Severe obesity, high blood pressure, and kidney problems—issues that landed me in the "underlying conditions" category, which I did not know about (other than me being overweight) prior to me getting infected—concerned the doctors. At that time, common practice was to place coronavirus patients on ventilators. Of those patients, studies were suggesting that patients placed on ventilators had a low survival rate.

So, there I was on this side of hell, preparing for the battle of my life. The doctors informed me that I would likely have to be put on a ventilator. My survival chances were not good. That is when I started getting scared. Amber had continued to text me trying to get an answer to her question. But my battery started running low.

Initially, I was thirsty, and they would not let me have anything to drink. The doctors gave me a pin code to give my family before they sedated me. The pin code allowed my family members to call the medical staff and inquire about my status. The pin code gave the doctors and nursing staff permission to disclose otherwise sensitive private information concerning my health. I had enough time before they were going to put me under to call Tiffany, who also tested positive for the coronavirus but was given an inhaler and allowed to go home. I made sure that she had Amber's phone number and the pin code, and asked her to make sure that she shared the code with Amber, and my father, because I figured I probably would be out of it later. Tiffany told me later that after I was sedated, she texted my father to tell him what was going on. He responded that he was on his way to Chicago. I do not think he ever made it, and it is probably best that he did not make it. They would not have allowed him into the hospital to see me anyway.

I had never been on a ventilator before, let alone had an extended stay at a hospital beyond the two days I spent in a hospital in Atlanta a month before I caught the coronavirus. Just the thought of that was scary. Initially, I was relieved when the doctors told me that "I looked like I was breathing better" and that they would hold off on putting me on the ventilator. I figured that was a sign that it was not as bad as it seemed. I have heard from people that work in hospitals that, in hindsight, I should have been treated with a CPAP machine and not a ventilator. Perhaps I should have refused to be placed on the ventilator, but I did not know any better. But to their credit, the U of C medical staff made me as comfortable as possible. I remember being moved to a regular room and watching TV. I remember talking with my mother on the phone and telling her that I tested positive for the virus. Later, I spoke with my brother Kris and told him as well. Kris started worrying that he might have to get tested. After all, Kris had a wife and three girls back at home. Fortunately, Kris tested negative and did not take the virus home with him. I remember watching one of the newer episodes of *NCIS: Los Angeles* on CBS, and the local Channel 2 News. At some point, I must have fallen asleep. After that, I do not remember anything. Apparently around 5:00am, the doctors called my mother, and informed her that I was suffering from pneumonia, and in order to make me comfortable, they sedated me and put me on the ventilator in the middle of the night.

CHAPTER 6

'So do not fear, for I am with you; do not be dismayed, for I am your GOD. I will strengthen you and help you; I will uphold you with my righteous right hand'

—Isaiah 41:10

After I was placed on a ventilator, I was sent to a new intensive care unit (ICU) that the hospital set up specifically for COVID-19 patients. The unit had a dedicated team of twelve medical professionals. As stated in the last chapter, on the first night I was in the hospital, doctors decided to put me on the ventilator after having trouble breathing overnight. It turns out I had pneumonia and my blood oxygen level was dipping too much too frequently. I wonder now if it could have been related to my undiagnosed sleep apnea at the time. Nevertheless, I was listed as critical, but stable condition. The decision was made to keep me on the ventilator until they felt I was getting adequate oxygen and my levels were stable. They kept me sedated and comfortable during all of this, so I was oblivious to everything that was going on. My life was no longer in my hands. My family and friends were forced to place their faith in GOD and acknowledge that only GOD had control and the power to pull me through. And GOD was going to pull me through.

The doctors gave me two antiviral agents that were recommended by the infectious control specialists. They also gave me antibiotics to treat my pneumonia. They placed a central line into my blood vessel to allow for the medication to treat my low blood pressure. This ultimately caused blood clots in my hand, which I will discuss later. They also discovered that I had a problem with my kidneys, which they deduced was created by the virus. In general, doctors were seeing kidney and liver issues developing in coronavirus patients. At the time, my kidney issues improved due to the fluids they were giving me, and I could produce my own urine. The doctors estimated that I would only be in the hospital for two weeks.

Not much changed over the next few days. I remained under sedation and on the ventilator, while my blood pressure and oxygen levels remained stable. But the darker color of my urine indicated the virus was attacking my kidneys. The doctors had to decide within 24 hours whether to put me on dialysis. Had I been awake, that would have scared me. My best friend, Otha Smith, had to go through years of dialysis before he had his kidney transplant in 2014.

Thinking back, I believe this was when I started having hallucinations in the form of dreams. A couple of times, I dreamed that I was an old man in the hospital, refusing to be taken off the ventilator because I was waiting on somebody. I remember seeing the TV screen menu in my hospital room. So, I know that to some degree, I was conscious while sedated. I also remember having dreams during the moments I was being shifted from bed to bed, transported via the elevators, and remember hearing the staff members discussing their after-work plans.

For the first few days, there was no real change in my condition, and no signs that the virus had regressed. My family and friends remained prayerful. This was a battle for GOD to handle, and it was just getting started.

On day seven, the doctors reported that I was doing great and breathing mostly on my own. The virus was still attacking my kidney function. Thus they continued to monitor the color of my urine, but all my electrolytes looked good. At the time, they initially determined that I would not need dialysis. They were considering taking me off the ventilator. The next day, the doctors were incredibly pleased with my progress. The doctors were also happy to report to my mother that I was starting to rely less on the ventilator. They also reported that I was starting to wake up and squeezing the doctor's hand on request—that part I do remember. My blood pressure returned to my usual hypertensive level, and thus, they started giving me the meds that I had previously been prescribed prior to contracting the coronavirus.

The next day, the doctors feared that I suffered a stroke. As the sedation started to wear off, I was not responding as

I should. But my lungs looked good and I was continuing to produce my own urine. The CT scan came back negative. This was probably the most stressful day for my mother throughout this process. Here I was, several days in the hospital. At the time, they were not allowing any outside visitors into the hospital. It was at this point that my mother asked the doctors if they thought I would survive. The doctors told my mother that, while they certainly could not make any guarantees, I was young and strong enough to make it through this and survive. My mother then told the doctors that she was 67 years old, that I was her only child, and she was not going to have any other children—she asked them to do whatever was necessary to save me.

Twelve days after being admitted to the hospital, the doctor called my mother at 5:30am for permission to perform a blood transfusion. My blood pressure was dropping, and my white cell count was off. She gave them permission for the blood transfusion, and for them to proceed with dialysis, which they had originally hoped to avoid. They also found a blood clot in my leg, which raised more concern, especially since my grandfather, Ceroy Hollis, had died twenty-nine years earlier from a similar blood clot in his leg. This obviously worried my mother. I even recall my stepfather having issues with blood clots in his leg at some point while in his 40s or 50s. Additionally, they found evidence of internal bleeding. Even though the doctors had initially taken me off the ventilator, my condition had worsened, and so they decided to put me back on the ventilator later that day. They then scheduled another CT scan, and prepared me for dialysis.

The next day, they began putting me on dialysis. They believed that this was a temporary measure. The doctors hoped that this would help alleviate some of the confusion I experienced when I was awake, as well as improve my kidney fluids. I ended up receiving a second blood transfusion. This time, it appeared to be working as my blood count and blood pressure began to stabilize. A CT scan was performed both on my chest and abdomen, and they identified two sources of internal bleeding—one in my back, and the other in my abdomen. I had an intervention team that was monitoring me the whole time. They determined that despite identifying the bleeding sources, nothing other than continued monitoring was required at the time. They also stopped giving me the medication for the blood clot in my leg to hopefully promote internal healing. As a precaution, they again sedated me and placed me back on the ventilator to keep me comfortable and keep my heart rate stable. They continued giving me antibiotics to try to prevent infection. All in all, the doctors felt I was more stable on day thirteen, than I was on day twelve.

I had been a fighter all my life. I fought to get my high school diploma by delivering a paper to my senior English teacher the night of my senior prom. I fought my way into law school and graduated after taking a year off during law school. I had to take the Illinois Bar exam seven times before I finally passed and became a licensed attorney. Fighting is what I do. And now, with the biggest battle of my life ahead of me, maybe even subconsciously, I was not about to stop now, or go quietly without a fight. Somewhere deep down inside, I knew I was going to fight off this virus. Indeed, I was fighting and starting to win the battle. I was not going to let my daughters down, especially Amber, nor have my grand-baby grow up without at least having the chance of seeing or knowing her grandfather, nor was I going to let my parents bury me. As Amber stated in one of her text messages to me, I had to live, and I had to survive and beat this thing. It was going to take a miracle, but in no way was I done living yet.

CHAPTER 7

'I will say of the LORD, "He is my refuge and my fortress, my GOD, in whom I trust." Surely, he will save you from the fowler's snare and from the deadly pestilence. He will cover you with his feathers, and under his wings you will find refuge; his faithfulness will be your shield and rampart'

– Psalm 91:1

On Day 14, the doctors were happy to provide a better report to my mother and Amber. They took me off sedation and removed the breathing tube, and I was finally breathing independently. The medical staff asked me how I felt, and I remember whispering "ok" to one of the nurses. That was apparently my first coherent response since I was first sedated. I remember, as I was waking up out of sedation, the nurse was wiping my mouth with what tasted like toothpaste. Ironically, my two favorite movies, *"CAPTAIN MARVEL"* and *"THE AVENGERS: END GAME,"* were on the TV. This was really the first time that I was conscious of the fact that I was still in the hospital. Soon after I woke up, one of the nurses came in and told me that I had a phone call. They put the phone up to my ear, I was very weak and very tired and could not hold it on my own. But I mustered up enough energy to say "Hello?"

All I heard were two excited voices from two women screaming "HAAAAAY!!" —I had no idea who it was.

One of the voices asked, "Do you know who this is?" Deliriously, I asked if they were my sisters. Then, one of the voices said, "he thinks we are his sisters." At that point I recognized that voice—it was Karen, which meant the other voice had to be Amber. I was immediately in tears. It was the first time they had heard my voice since I had been in the hospital. And I was so happy to hear their voices as well. Later that same day, I received a call from Tiffany and my mother. Tiffany screamed out "Oh my GOD, we have been praying for you", as she started naming her friends and classmates that had reached out to her asking how I was doing. My mother just kept telling me "you have truly been blessed." It was not until two weeks later, after I had been moved out of ICU, that I powered on my phone and saw all the text messages from Amber, urging me to fight this virus and wake up, and her heartbreaking messages chronicling her feelings of helplessness while I was sedated. I also laughed as I read her texts about how Karen went into "super mom mode" and went off on a nursing staff member after they had pissed them both off somehow. I also read how she, Amber, called the hospital staff every single day while I was under sedation, how scared she was and that she could not stop crying.

Before heading to the hospital, I did not really get a chance to tell Amber what was wrong with me. But Amber, second only to my mother and Tiffany, was indeed my biggest prayer warrior. Amber's text messages were almost like her own personal journal to me, which shed some light on everything I went through while I was sedated and on the ventilator. She was so scared that I would not pull through. Amber also texted several times that she loved me. I could tell from her text messages when she grew confident in the fact that I would be okay, and that I was getting better. It was as if she knew that GOD was going to pull me through.

I was still on the dialysis machine, my blood pressure was high when I was breathing, and I still had a blood clot in my leg. The doctors did not want to take the risk of putting me on a blood thinner yet because I still had internal bleeding and they were concerned about the clot moving to my lungs or heart. Although I was not out of the woods yet, it was clear that all the prayers were starting to be answered and that GOD was pulling me through this ordeal. Despite the insurmountable odds, there was proof that I was a living miracle, and that I was not done living yet.

As the days went by, I became more engaged with the doctor. I was told I laughed at his jokes (what I remember saying to him was: "you have jokes"). I was breathing with extraordinarily little oxygen support. I remained on dialysis, but I was beginning to make my own urine. The blood clots still remained a major concern. My hand specialist, Dr. Jennifer Wolf, provided some recommendations based on the numbness I had in my thumb, index finger, and pinky, indicating that a blood clot was impacting blood flow. The other concern was the blood clot in my leg. The medical staff balanced the risk of giving me a blood thinner, which could cause more internal bleeding versus the possible dislodging of a clot into my lungs. Nevertheless, I was in a much better place than I was four days prior.

On Friday April 3rd, 2020, they began to transition me off dialysis. My breathing and oxygenation were good. My blood pressure and blood counts remained stable. They started treating me with anti-coagulation drugs to dissolve the blood clot in my leg—treatment used to prevent the formation of new blood clots, prevent current blood clots from growing in size, and reduce the risk of embolization of existing clots into vital organs such as the lungs. Barring any unforeseen surprises, the medical staff prepared to move me out of ICU into a regular room the next day.

On Saturday, April 4th, 2020 I was finally off both the ventilator and dialysis. I was awake and finally being discharged—or so I thought. I was merely being transferred out of ICU into a regular room. Although that was a good thing, I was pissed because I thought I was going home. Nevertheless, being moved out of ICU meant I was one step closer to going home. I did not require any oxygen, which meant my breathing was good. I had a speech pathologist come visit me several times to assess my ability to eat. At first, she determined that I could only eat soft foods, but later, cleared me for a regular diet. I was a difficult patient to deal with once I got out of ICU. I was frustrated because I no longer wanted to be in the hospital. I could not do anything. I think I watched every single *Madea* movie, and every episode of *College Hill* that came on BET. I even watched numerous press briefings by President Donald Trump, which continued to prove that he had mishandled the country's response to the pandemic.

I particularly was not happy with the food choices they were trying to feed me. I do not eat eggs—anyone who knows me knows that. The smell of eggs makes me gag. The first day out of ICU, one of the male nurses shoved some eggs down my throat. I threw them up. One of the doctors then called my mother and had her speak to me to reiterate that if I did not eat, I would not regain my strength and I might not make it out of the hospital. I told her, as well as the doctor later, that I do not have a problem eating. I just did not like the food that they were trying to force feed me. So, I made a deal with the doctor to let me order what I want to eat every day off the hospital menu, and we would have no problem with me eating. The doctor agreed and we had no problems after that. The food was still dry most days, but I could order multiple fruit cups, red jello, Ensure protein drink (which I still drink now), lemonade, and similar favorite foods of mine.

My memory was starting to come back, even though there was still some confusion. Somehow before I left ICU, I managed to pull out both my feeding tube and my dialysis catheter cap. I do not remember any of that, but it is certainly possible. My kidney numbers were still unstable. However, they were improving with each passing day. The doctors saw no reason for me to be placed on emergency dialysis. But it meant that my blood had to be drawn every day. Every morning, the phlebotomist would wake me up early in the morning, always wanting to find a vein in my hand. I did not mind my arm because I did not feel it as bad. But I felt pain in my hand, and I was very irritable. If they missed the vein on the first try, I would refuse to allow them to stick the needle in me again without finding someone else who could do it.

I was still on anticoagulants for the blood clots. There was no further evidence of internal bleeding, and my blood pressure was normal. The expectation was that I would be in the hospital for another week or two, and then I would be transferred to an acute rehabilitation center primarily to help me learn how to walk again. The challenge I faced was that my legs were not strong enough, and given the time I spent on the ventilator, I was unable to walk when I first woke up out of sedation. I had two physical therapists visit me daily to help me to start walking again. My initial rehab was limited to my hotel room because they were not allowing patients to access the hallways at that time. First, I had to learn how to stand on my own, then continue standing for a period of time. Then, with help, after standing, I had to re-learn how to walk from the bed to either the sofa or the chair that was in my room. They wanted me to spend at least an hour sitting up in the chair; they said it was better for my lungs.

One day, after I had sat in the chair for over an hour, I called the nurse as instructed to help me back to the bed. The nurse assigned to me was mean as hell. I believe her name was Michelle. She would not let me go back to bed until after lunch. I was angry because the nurse was not listening to me, or my physical therapist. At first, I argued with her and told her what my physical therapists said, but she did not care and was not going to help me. I felt hopeless—I was at the mercy of a nurse that did not realize who the f*ck I was. I thought to myself, 'I'm Big Daddy Esquire! I can do this myself". I finally just said f*ck it and found a way to get into bed myself.

Finding a rehab center that accepted COVID-19 patients was another challenge I faced. The preferred rehab center, Ingalls Rehabilitation Center, would not accept me until my kidney numbers were stable, and I had to get two negative COVID-19 tests before they could transport me to rehab. That just added to my impatience and desire to get the f*ck out of the hospital. Not to mention, I had forgotten how irritating the tests were—sticking a q-tip way up my nose. Talking to Amber everyday calmed me down a bit. We later laughed about me asking to go home as soon as I woke up from being sedated in the ICU.

Eventually, I found my phone in my bag of clothes. One of the nurses agreed to charge it for me. Once I finally had a fully charged phone, I logged onto Facebook for the first time in nearly a month, to let everyone know that I did not fall off the face of the Earth, I was doing better, and looking forward to getting out of the hospital soon. My post ended up with over 500 likes and nearly just as many words of encouragement. I also spoke to Kris and Abdullah, Tiffany, Terri my paralegal, and Curtis, my best friend since we were young, almost daily. I told Curtis how hurt and disappointed I was that I did not hear from my daughter Vivian. She had not texted or called me once since being in the hospital. He told me not to worry about that right now, and just focus on getting better, and continue to foster and enjoy my relationship with Amber. That I had done all I could do up to that point, and advised that I should leave the door open for Vivian to come back and rebuild our relationship when she was ready.

On April 17th, 2020, my kidney numbers finally lowered below the required level to allow the hospital to release and transport me to the rehab center. Additionally, both my COVID-19 tests came back negative. I was so excited and ready—I was finally going to Ingalls Rehabilitation Center in Harvey, Illinois, one step before finally going home. While I was waiting on the transport vehicle in my room, with my clothes packed and ready to go, I sat on the sofa and reflected on everything I had been through (that I was aware of) during my stay at U of C hospital. I cried for a moment, because I knew that I was only still alive solely by the grace of GOD. Before I left, the doctor came in to speak to me about making sure I took better care of myself. His exact words were, "You were lucky this time around. But if lighting strikes a second time, you may not be as fortunate." I heard what he said and was determined to adopt a new attitude once I could go home. Before long, 2pm had arrived, the transport ambulance was due to arrive and transport me to rehab. I was ready to go. They loaded me on a transport bed—it hurt like hell. But I did not care. I was about to "blow this popsicle stand" and leave the hospital. I was one step closer to going home. As the transport folks wheeled me out of my room and out to the elevators, I said goodbye to the nursing staff that I had become cool with. After that, I was transported by ambulance out of the University of Chicago hospital to Ingalls in Harvey, Illinois.

I arrived at Ingalls at around 3pm in the afternoon. By the time I had arrived, my mother had already dropped off a bag of clean clothes, sweatshirts, pants, socks and a phone charger that Tiffany had purchased for me. My mom also brought the notebook I asked her to bring so that I could start writing notes for the book. I did not want to forget any parts of my story. It was not until I got to rehab, that my mother forwarded me all the text messages she sent out almost daily to update my friends and family regarding my health. When I read the text messages, I was shocked. I could not believe it. I went through all of that? It finally became clear to me why everyone I spoke to kept telling me that I was blessed, and a miracle. How is it possible that I am still here—still living? I was overcome with emotion. But I got myself together, and just kept thanking GOD that I made it to rehab.

Unlike at the hospital, where I had my own room, I shared a room with Mr. Ernest at Ingalls. Mr. Ernest was an older gentleman, who had also been hospitalized at the University of Chicago (Harvey Campus) with the coronavirus.

I think he had been at Ingalls for about a week prior to my arrival. Around 3:30pm, a lady from the kitchen staff came around and took our Saturday breakfast, lunch, and dinner orders. I ate great on that first day. I had pancakes, grits, bacon and sausage for breakfast, a cheeseburger for lunch, and Salisbury steak for dinner—by far the best meals I had in a while, and way better than any of the meals I had while in the hospital. We did not get a chance to order any meals for Sunday and boy did it make a helluva difference. The meals on Sunday left a lot to be desired. They served milk with every meal—milk! I had several cans of generic ginger ale and cola to drink. Later, I figured out how to order things via UberEATS, grub hub, and door dash.

The first day of rehab was the Monday after I arrived. That is when I met Kevin Vicari, my primary physical therapist (PT). Kevin was a cool white guy. I told him that my goal was to get out of there and get back to work ASAP. I told him that he should feel free to put me through the rigors of physical therapy. That first day, we went outside for the first time since I was admitted to the ER. I did not realize how much I had missed the smell of fresh air. I walked up and down the stairs, and through the parking lot. First with a walker, but later with Kevin just holding a belt that was wrapped around my waist so I would not fall. Soon, I was walking on my own. However, there was concern about me going back home because, at the time, I lived in a one-bedroom apartment on the third floor of my building.

Also, on that first day, I met Teri, my occupational therapist (OT)—ironically, she had the same name as my paralegal. She helped me wash up, brush my teeth, tie my shoes, and put on my underwear. I had not really followed the rules whenever I wanted to go to the bathroom, and/or take a shower—the presence of a nurse was always required for such activities. Look, I was just excited to even take a shower for the first time in a month. After having to pee through a catheter, or in a urinal (after the catheter was removed), poop in a bed pan, and have my ass wiped in bed, you would be ready and happy to take a shower as well and would not give a damn about following the rules either. That was the most humiliating part of this ordeal. I also had not had a haircut in a month, and was looking very grizzly, as if I had been on another sabbatical.

I spent about eleven days total in rehab. I was not supposed to be released until May 5th, 2020. But I put my head down and put in the work—six hours a day—while I was there. Then on April 28th, 2020, my care coordinator told me that the doctors and rehab staff reviewed my overall progress and felt comfortable sending me home, and that if I wanted to, I could go home the next day. FINALLY!! I yelled out when I heard the amazing news. I was finally ready to go home. I called my mother to make sure she was available to pick me up the next day. Later that same day, I worked with another therapist named Dean. He and I walked underneath the tunnel from the rehab center, up the stairs, and across the street (underground) to the hospital. That apparently was my last test to make sure I was fit to go home. We went to the cafeteria, where he bought me a grape soda. After that, we sat in one of the reception areas, chopped it up for about thirty minutes, and then walked across the street, and back to the Rehab center. That night I could not sleep. I was too excited about going home the next day. I stayed up watching my favorite show *Chicago PD* on USA until about 5am. Just before I went to sleep, I posted a picture of my room from the bed, and this message below on Facebook:

Dear Lord:

I'm going home today. I never thought I would say that again two months ago. I miss my family. I can't wait to see them today. And I owe that to you. Thank you for standing side-by-side with me as I went into battle with the coronavirus. Thank you for bringing me out on the other side. Thank you for blessing me with the greatest mother I could've ever asked for. Thank you for surrounding me with the medical and rehab professionals you have surrounded me with. Most of all, thank you for giving me a second chance at living again.

In Jesus name
Amen
#iaintdonelivingyet
492 likes
135 comments
7 shares

I woke up just in time for breakfast at 8:30am and completed my last day of physical therapy. My mother and stepfather arrived at around 11:30am. It was the first time I had seen my mother since I was hospitalized because no visitors were allowed due to coronavirus protocols. When I saw my mother, I immediately hugged her. I was overwhelmed with tears and emotion. My mother made several visits, delivering clean clothes to the hospital staff to give to me. Kris came twice, once to bring me Harold's Chicken, and the second time to bring my keys and my other cell phone that was buried in my bed. Tiffany was kind enough to bring me some KFC, but would not let me order anything that was not grilled. And Terri, my paralegal, was kind enough to bring me my laptop bag. The rehab staff often commented on how I was the only patient working in the hospital. They did not understand that I was there to get back to work—Period!

By 12:00pm, I was discharged from rehab and finally on my way home. Before I left, I made sure to say goodbye to Kevin and Teri and thanked them for everything, while I was in rehab. That night, from my office/den at home, I got on Facebook Live, and thanked everyone for all the prayers and well wishes. It was the first time that many had seen my face in two months. I called my barber, Ahz, and set up an appointment with him two days later, to finally get a fresh cut. Everyone was so worried about me catching the virus again from a haircut, and whether Ahz was properly sanitizing his cutting tools and cleaning areas, especially Amber. But Ahz graciously assured her that he was sanitizing everything and taking all the proper precautions. I was so happy to get that grizzly look taken care of.

CHAPTER 8

'Today is the day that the Lord has made.
Let us rejoice and be glad in it'

—Psalm 118:24

Even during all this chaos, GOD still has a way of letting you know that He cares about you and all your needs. Shortly after getting out of the hospital, I was able to purchase a 2016 Ford Explorer. It was needed because it helped me resolve another problem that had been lingering for some time. I had a 2014 Black Cadillac ATS that I was having difficulty getting in and out of, and I needed an SUV. So, you can say it was a 'grateful-to-GOD-I'm-alive purchase', but for me, it was another prayer that had been answered. Being able to purchase this SUV assured me that GOD was giving me all the tools I needed to live a normal life after my COVID-19 experience. And if I did not know then that GOD had a special plan for my life, it was starting to become clear with each passing day. But the road to recovery was certainly not over.

On May 11th, 2020, I met with my orthopedic hand specialist. The clots that developed in my hand made the tips of my right index finger and thumb pitch black and extremely painful. I was able to type without any problems, but my handwriting and signature were very shaky. During my appointment, Dr. Wolf examined my hand and allowed me to wrap it for the first time since I developed the clots. My hand was being treated with Nitroglycerin—a treatment cream commonly used for heart patients. Dr. Wolf wanted to wait at least two months before having to decide whether to amputate the tips of my finger and thumb. As the days went by, the pain increased, and it honestly never got better.

On May 28th, 2020, after one of my occupational therapy sessions at the University of Chicago medical facility in Flossmoor, Illinois, I posted images of the damage the blood clots had done to my hand on social media. For the most part, the response was met with more prayers for healing and well wishes. But a nurse from Orlando, Florida, posted a comment trying to discredit what I shared by stating that my symptoms were not related to COVID-19. She claimed that she has been a nurse for 18 years, and a COVID-19 liaison for the same amount of time at her hospital in Orlando. But she is not a doctor.

At first, I did not see her comment. I just noticed that my friends were jumping on her case. When I finally went back to read her comments, I was both outraged and hurt that someone would call me a liar after everything I had been through. On the other hand, I took this as an opportunity to educate her, and others, on how I got the clots in my hand, including what my doctor said as well. Nevertheless, I was still troubled by her response. It took a lot for me to share my story of battling the coronavirus with everyone, and for this person, someone I do not know from a can of paint, to call me a liar on social media, was too much to handle. I canceled my rehab appointment that was scheduled two days later, and I did not go back to the office the rest of the week. I just needed a mental break.

That following Thursday, I posted a message thanking everyone who had been supportive of me sharing my story on social media. I let everyone know that this individual was blocked from my Facebook page because she clearly had an agenda to stir up some mess. I also reminded folks that for whatever reason, GOD gave me a second chance at life to tell my story. And as the State of Illinois was preparing to re-open the government, retail businesses, barbershops, beauty salons, and open restaurants for outdoor dining, I was reminded that life must move on, and we should too. This virus has not gone away, but you got to keep living.

I stressed the importance that we take precautions, but not stop living. What I meant by that was to continue to wear masks, maintain a social distance of at least six feet apart, and most importantly—wash your hands for at least 20 seconds. But do not stop living your life. Continue to travel and do everything you were doing before the pandemic. When our number is called, that is when it is time to go be with GOD. That is when you stop living, but until then, it is important to enjoy life.

On June 3rd, 2020, I met with Dr. Wolf, to re-examine my hand. I told her how it felt like whatever was underneath the blackened tips of my index finger was pushing upward—trying to break free. It was so painful that I told her that if my quality of life would be improved going forward, I would prefer that she go ahead and schedule the amputation procedure. It just so happened that the next available date was June 4th, 2020, the next day. I did not think the surgery would happen that soon. However, I wanted to get it over with, and start the healing process. Of course, that meant taking another coronavirus test—the irritating sticking of the q-tip *waaaay* up my nose—my sixth test since being released from the hospital. Man, I hated that test. The test came back negative. I was relieved, but saddened at the thought of my fingers being cut off. But I knew it had to be done, and ultimately made peace with that. The surgery was scheduled for 2pm the next day.

The next day, I had an emergency court hearing that morning on a guardianship matter I was handling. That took my mind off things temporarily. But I was extremely nervous about having part of my fingers removed. But once again, GOD had given me a sense of comfort. My anesthesiologist, Dr. Kurtz, remembered me from the ICU when I had the coronavirus, and he made me feel comfortable because he was familiar with me. There was also a nurse who kept my spirits up. Unfortunately, I do not remember her name, but I am thankful that she was there to prep me during my pre-op. Later that day, I had the surgery to amputate the tips of my right thumb and index finger. I cannot remember much about this procedure outside of being very thirsty because I could not eat or drink anything all day before my procedure. So, I prepared for this and brought a bottle of orange Gatorade in my bag to drink after the surgery was over. I told everyone that I wanted my Gatorade as soon as I got out of surgery. Luckily, as I was waking up after the surgery, the surgical staff spoke to my mother. She specifically reminded them that I had a bottle of Gatorade in my bag that I wanted to have post-surgery.

After leaving the hospital, and getting my prescription for Oxycodone, I returned home. When I got there, Tiffany, my dad, and Kyra (my law office partner) were there waiting on me. My dad, 69 years old at the time, and a high risk to the virus, drove four hours to Chicago from suburban Detroit, just to be there and lay eyes on me. My dad said that he needed to see for himself that I was okay. He stayed until midnight, and then, got on the road and headed back to Detroit. Meanwhile, back at home, I rested comfortably for the rest of the evening. I ate that good food that Kyra had brought over. Though my arm was still numb, I was not feeling any pain. That was until 4am, when the numbness wore off. I woke up from my sleep, hollering, and in intense pain. Tylenol with Codeine was a lifesaver for the many painful nights to come. The Oxycodone just did NOT work.

Several weeks later, more than a month after the surgery, I started feeling depressed. I had been holding onto this façade that I was alright with parts of my fingers gone, but deep down inside, I was truly devastated. Slightly angry. My father had been anxiously trying to talk to me about 'being the chosen one' and comparing me to the story of Jacob. The story of Jacob, as it was told to me, involved Jacob wrestling with the angel that represented Jesus Christ. After the fight was over, GOD touched his hip so that he would remember the night he 'wrestled with the angel.' From that day on, Jacob walked with a limp. This made me think about the movie, *Remember the Titans,* when Coach Yost gave his defense the speech that I will always remember. "*You make sure that they remember, FOREVER, the night they played the Titans.*" According to my father, my amputated fingers was GOD's way of making sure I remembered what I went through with the coronavirus—not sure how I would ever forget those events.

Later that day, after the conversation, my father also texted me a picture of myself, with my mother, and my favorite aunt, Angela. Angela is eleven years older than me. So, in that picture, Angela had to be fourteen or fifteen, and I was about three or four years old. I know my father meant well, but that picture was hard for me to look at. Seeing myself as a boy, three or four years old, but having all my fingers back then was hard. Now, at forty-three, I have three and a half fingers on my right hand. I was incredibly sad, and damn near inconsolable inside. But I kept my feelings private. The human in me asked: "Why Me?" At that point, it did not matter that I was the "walking miracle" after enduring what I went through. The truth is, this had been rough, and the mental strain had at times been unbearable. So, in private, I cried the tears I needed to cry, and pushed on. I have accepted that life goes on. I still had to work on the concept of moving on with life without all my fingers on my right hand. The way I have recovered from this ordeal is just yet another example of GOD's mercy and grace and was the answer to so many prayers by so many people.

About a week later, on my stepfather's and my mother's anniversary, Dr. Wolf sent me the article she co-wrote called: "*Digital Ischemia in COVID-19 Patients: Case Report*". The article discussed the origin of COVID-19 and critically ill patients with COVID-19 who developed extremity ischemia. The report referenced seven cases in Wuhan, China, critically ill patients with COVID pneumonia, five of which died from COVID related complications. The study went further to analyze two patients who were admitted to the emergency department at the University of Chicago hospital. Patient A was a 70-year-old woman who tested positive for COVID-19, with no known medical history—in a week, she experienced fevers, chills, worsening shortness breath, and headaches. Patient B was described as a 43-year-old male with a medical history of obesity, hypertension, shortness of breath, cough, and chest pain that had been progressively worsening over the past week, and reported fatigue, diarrhea and decreased urine output. Can you guess who Patient B was? You got it... yours truly, the author of this book, Marques A. Eason, Esq.

The article went on to discuss how within 24 hours of being admitted to the emergency room, I tested positive for the virus and demonstrated worsening breathing issues, which required them to transfer me to the ICU and intubate me. The report also displayed pictures of my right hand, which included the tips of my index finger and thumb, both of which were blackened due to blood clots. The report highlighted how I was initially treated with the blood thinner, Heparin, but later transitioned to "apixaban 5 mg" (otherwise known as *Eliquis*), which I am currently still taking now. For Patient B, the report stated that 'ultimately, the patient was discharged to an acute care rehabilitation facility after sufficient clinical recovery'. For Patient A, however, the decision was made to pursue comfort care (otherwise known as "hospice") and the patient ultimately died.

That was beyond heavy for me. It should be no surprise that I was overly emotional when I read this report. I immediately called my mother and told her that I had just read the report and I just did not understand. Why me? Why am I still here? Why did I survive when the 70-year-old woman with no known medical history did not make it? That's when she told me what she told the doctors about her being 67 years old, that I was her only son, and that she was not having any more children—they needed to do whatever it took to save me. I have a praying mother. And for whatever His reasons were, GOD answered her prayers and spared my life. I am forever thankful for my mother's courage, commitment, faith, and for the devotion to lift me up in prayer, and her refusal to let anyone give up on me.

FUTURE

'The key to making healthy decisions is to respect your future self. Honor him or her. Treat him or her like you would treat a friend or a loved one.'

A. J. Jacobs

CHAPTER 9

'You're not defined by your past;
you're prepared by it. You're stronger, more experienced,
and you have greater confidence'

—Joel Osteen

"Thy Will Be Done"

—Matthew 6:9-10

I was twenty-five years old the first time I heard Steve Harvey on his then local radio show in Los Angeles, California. Steve Harvey always started and ended his show by saying that 'GOD is everything and without GOD you ain't got nothing. You can believe that and take that to the bank', 'GOD is the answer to all things' and 'Prayer Changes Things.' I cried the first time I heard his show. Ever since that day, for the rest of my time in Los Angeles, I made sure that I was either up and, on my way to work, and/or had a radio on at 6:00am to listen to his morning sermon. That was my daily routine from 2002 to 2004.

In 2008, I bought tickets to Steve Harvey's comedy show in Atlanta, Georgia. I sat right in front, the fourth row from the stage. Again, at the end of the show, he gave honor to GOD and talked about how GOD is merciful and gracious, and how GOD can bring you from the back to the front. Many people judge Steve Harvey negatively, and thus, judged me for listening to him. Although I like Steve Harvey, my response was simple—who cares about the messenger. The point was, GOD used him as a vessel, or messenger, to make sure that I got what I needed to get out of his story. That was GOD's way of talking to me, reminding me that He, GOD, is always in control, He is the answer to all things, and that all things are possible through Him.

I can not help but sound like a broken record by saying again that I owe my life to GOD for bringing me back from the cusp of death, and giving me a second chance at living. GOD literally took me through hell, and brought me out, safe and sound, on the other side. The virus was wicked. It still is wicked. Had I been somewhere else, at another hospital in Chicago, other than the University of Chicago, or perhaps Northwestern University Hospital, I might not be sitting here sharing with everyone how lucky I am. I thank GOD in some way every day for sparing my life. He also blessed me, as he always has, by ensuring that I was financially set once I got back into the real world. I am blessed to still be able to live my dream, of being an attorney, and that it was not cut short at the age of forty-three. GOD gave me a second chance at life.

FATHER'S DAY 2020

On Father's Day, June 21st, 2020, I made a surprise trip to Atlanta, Georgia, to see Amber. I had been debating, going back and forth with myself about going all week mainly because I was concerned about whether the airlines were doing enough to protect its passengers. In fact, Amber, thinking she was not going to see me on Father's Day, had ordered three items off my Amazon Wish List—computer speakers, and two Apple Watch Bands (black and stainless steel). However, once I got on the plane, and saw how they separated us, and required all passengers to wear masks from the moment we boarded, I was fine. Karen pushed hard all week, urging me to come, citing that Amber needed to lay eyes on me. But just as important, I needed to lay eyes on her.

Karen and I stayed in communication while I was on the plane via text. We planned to meet at the Longhorn Steakhouse that was near the Atlanta airport, right off Camp Creek Parkway. Before taking off, Amber tried to Facetime me, presumably to wish me a Happy Father's Day. I did not answer because she would have figured out that I was on the plane and got suspicious. When I arrived at Atlanta's Hartsfield International Airport, I picked up a rental car and texted Karen to let her know I was on my way to Longhorn.

When I arrived, I parked in the back of the restaurant to make sure that Amber could not see me through any windows. Karen had already informed me that they were sitting at the bar. Karen had Amber save a seat, telling her that it was for her friend Tamika (Tamika was never coming, it was just me). When I walked into the restaurant, Amber was sitting at the bar with her back turned. I quickly walked behind her and said, "Excuse me, is this seat taken?" She initially looked at me in disbelief, as if she were dreaming, and was not really sure if I was standing there. When it finally settled in that it was not a dream, that I was standing there, she fell into my arms, wrapped her arms around my neck, and just started crying. Then, I started crying and kissed her on the forehead. The look on her face was like a photo that needed no words. I had finally got to see my baby, lay eyes on her, and let her see for herself that I was okay. Many people felt that I risked exposure to the virus again by traveling to Atlanta. But I did not care. There was absolutely nothing that anyone could do to keep me from seeing my baby on Father's Day. It was well worth the trip—and the best Father's Day gift ever.

HOPEFUL

As we stand here today, Coronavirus cases are spiking in the U.S. People need to take heed to the warnings from local government officials. The vaccines are coming, but we need to get there because this pandemic is not anywhere close to being over. There is no rhyme or reason as to how the virus will impact you. Just please protect yourself to the best extent possible. I don't wish what I went through on my worst enemy. I love my daughter Amber; she is a stone-cold soldier.

I love and miss my daughter Vivian, and my granddaughter Blake, very much. But it is what it is right now. I dream of all of us being together one day—a dream that I believe will come true one day.

As I work through my story in this book, mentally and physically, I look forward to the day when I can completely get this stuff off my chest and share it with all of you. It has been therapeutic for me to share bits and pieces of my story with so many. And I am so thankful that, for the most part, everyone has embraced me telling my story. I feel like part of that is my purpose for still being alive. By writing this book, I wanted to give a real-life example of the damage that the coronavirus can cause to an individual, to encourage self-education and awareness of the coronavirus, and to testify as a living, breathing witness to yet another one of GOD's miracles. I can not express thoroughly how grateful I am that GOD spared my life in sparing my life and let me live another day.

I want to fulfill my destiny, and purpose—whatever that may be. Hopefully, I will have at least another forty to fifty years, if not more, to live the dream I am living right now. I have launched a new campaign for my law firm—a new website that has also captured the story of my battle with the coronavirus. I have a new outlook on life overall. I appreciate things more than I probably did before my near-death experience. I know my mother is happy because about not having to hear constant bickering from me regarding the things that upset me before with my stepfather. I have realized that I am blessed, and life is too short to not choose my battles wisely. Plus, I'm thankful that Irv, my stepfather, stood with my mother while she was trying to hold it together as I battled the virus.

I cannot thank GOD enough for blessing my life ten times over, and for surrounding me with the people that he has surrounded me with, namely my mother, and especially that angel in the Sky looking after me, who we (CREW) all know and love simply as "O". I cannot explain it because it does not always make sense to me. What I do understand, as Joel Osteen accurately described is that; GOD had a purpose for taking me through this battle with the coronavirus. In this shaking, GOD shifted me into a new position. Opportunities will come before me that I would not have been ready for had there not been this shifting that GOD made happen in my life. The miracle is already in motion. GOD is up to something big. This pandemic did not happen by mistake. This is GOD's calling to find out who among us are true believers. I am a true believer. All good things come from GOD. I believe some blessings will come to all of us—especially me. The shaking is a sign that GOD is shifting things in favor of those who believe in Him.

Despite the progress I have made in my recovery, I still have a long way to go, but I am taking great strides to live and eat better, and enjoy the blessings that GOD continues to provide. I still struggle with my breathing, and recently bought an elliptical machine to help improve my overall breathing.

At times I find it difficult to speak for long periods of time. I no longer drink alcohol as much as I used to—maybe one to two drinks a week. I am trying to do things the right way and show GOD that I appreciate the life He has given me, and the second chance to live my life, pursue my dreams, and fulfill whatever purpose He has laid out for me. Most importantly, I get to tell the world, or anyone who will listen, that even when it appears as if the chips are stacked against you, when you least expect it, GOD will show up and show out for you. I am living proof of that. I am GOD's example that if you believe in him, keep him first in your life, stay on faith street, and stay prayerful, he will make it alright in the end. I have no business being on this Earth right now, but GOD has this amazing thing called mercy and grace, and you are never too far gone for Him to come back and get you—if you want him too.

With that said, I hope everyone reading this book learned something and has benefitted from me sharing my story. As a country, and as one of many nations, we have a lot of work to do during this pandemic before it ends. The coronavirus knows no color or gender. Eventually, we will get through this pandemic, once and for all. But until then, please protect yourselves by wearing masks, adhere to social distancing guidelines, wash your hands, and take other precautions that health experts have mandated as necessary to get through this pandemic. We serve a supernatural GOD who is not limited by the things we are limited by. What's impossible to people, is always possible with GOD. This pandemic did not happen by accident. On the surface, the shaking appeared like it was a negative thing. But without it, GOD clearly felt that I would not fulfill his purpose for me.

I thank GOD for blessing me and only hope that I can be a blessing to someone else. I thank GOD for shaking me and shifting me into a position of favor. Through all the things that one in my position would worry about—after not having worked for two months and recovering from a life-threatening experience as I have—GOD has shown me that I have nothing to worry about. He has made sure, through his blessings, that I would have everything I needed upon my re-entry into this new world as we know it.

Through this pandemic, and my experience, I have learned about the power of prayer. I have learned the importance of always staying prayerful, no matter what, watching GOD show up and show out for me. My hope is that the spiritual lessons learned throughout this ordeal will encourage all of you to stay prayerful, watch how the power of GOD will manifest itself, and how GOD will launch you to a new level and show you unprecedented favor, just as He has shown me in such a short time during my recovery from my battle with the coronavirus. One touch of His favor will catapult you into a new position of favor.

Not a day goes by that I am not thankful to still be on this Earth—after so many others have succumbed and passed away due to this deadly virus. There is no question that GOD has a purpose for me and there is a reason why he made me a living miracle. I do not take lightly that there are others, i.e., Gregg Garfield ("patient zero") whose story of survival is far more amazing and miraculous than mine.[8] May GOD continue to bless all of us, during this time of uncertainty. May GOD continue to show all of us great favor. May GOD continue to bless all the families who have lost loved ones during this pandemic. May GOD continue to bless all of us during this unprecedented coronavirus pandemic. May GOD continue to bless me and demonstrate his favor through me to all who I come in contact with and allow me to demonstrate further why *I Ain't Done Living Yet!!*

---

8   Gregg Garfield, known as Patient Zero, tested positive for the coronavirus on March 5th, 2020 in Los Angeles, California, after a ski trip to Italy with 13 others. All 13 caught the virus, but Gregg's health became worse over time. He was in hospital for 64 days—41 days on a ventilator.

www.ingramcontent.com/pod-product-compliance
Lightning Source LLC
Chambersburg PA
CBHW050733030426
42336CB00012B/1543